Dietary Therapies for Digestive Health: A Clinician's Handbook

Proven Nutritional Strategies for IBS, GERD, IBD, and Optimal Gut Health

By

Dr. M. Qassim

Aug. 2024

Table of Contents:

Introduction:

Welcome to "Dietary Therapies for Digestive Health: A Clinician's Handbook." In an era where chronic digestive disorders are becoming increasingly prevalent, the importance of understanding the intricate relationship between diet and digestive health cannot be overstated. This book is crafted to serve as a comprehensive guide for clinicians, nutritionists, and health enthusiasts who are keen on exploring the profound impact that nutrition can have on digestive health.

I.   Why This Book?

Digestive health is a cornerstone of overall well-being. A healthy digestive system not only ensures optimal nutrient absorption but also plays digestive disorders such as irritable bowel syndrome(IBS), Gastroesophageal Reflux Disease (GERD), Inflammatory Bowel Disease (IBD), and various other conditions. This book aims to provide a detailed exploration of how targeted dietary interventions can be used to manage and alleviate these conditions effectively.

II.   The Scope of the Book:

"Dietary Therapies for Digestive Health: A Clinician's Handbook" is divided into 15 chapters, each meticulously designed to cover a wide range of topics crucial for understanding and improving digestive health through nutrition. From understanding the basics of the digestive system and the gut microbiome to exploring specific dietary strategies for common digestive disorders, this book offers a holistic approach to digestive health.

You will find in-depth discussions on the role of fiber, hydration, fermented foods, and functional foods in promoting digestive wellness. Additionally, this handbook addresses the gut-brain connection, emphasizing how nutrition can support mental health, and provides practical strategies for managing digestive health across different life stages, including for children and the elderly.

III.   Practical and Evidence-Based:

This handbook is not just theoretical; it is deeply rooted in clinical practice and real-life applications. Each chapter includes evidence-based strategies, practical tips, and easy-to-follow meal plans and recipes that can be implemented in daily life. You will also find real-life case studies and success stories that illustrate the transformative power of dietary therapies in managing digestive health.

IV.   For Whom is This Book?

Whether you are a healthcare professional seeking to enhance your knowledge and practice, a nutritionist looking for practical tools and strategies, or an individual struggling with digestive issues and seeking effective solutions, this book is for you. It is designed to be a valuable resource that bridges the gap between scientific research and practical application, making complex nutritional concepts accessible and actionable.

V.   My Goal:

My goal with this handbook is to empower you with the knowledge and tools necessary to take control of digestive health through dietary interventions. By understanding the underlying mechanisms of how specific foods and nutrients impact the digestive system, you can make informed decisions that promote healing, prevent disease, and enhance overall well-being.

As you embark on this journey through the pages of "Dietary Therapies for Digestive Health: A Clinician's Handbook," we encourage you to approach the material with an open mind and a willingness to integrate new strategies into your practice or personal health regimen. Together, we can unlock the potential of dietary therapies to transform digestive health and improve quality of life.

Welcome to a new era of understanding and managing digestive health through the power of nutrition. Let's begin this journey toward optimal digestive wellness.

Chapter 1
Introduction to Digestive Health

I.   <u>Overview of the Digestive System:</u>

The digestive system is a complex network of organs and processes that work together to convert food into energy and essential nutrients needed for the body's functions. This intricate system includes the mouth, esophagus, stomach, small intestine, large intestine (colon), rectum, and anus. Accessory organs such as the liver, pancreas, and gallbladder also play critical roles in digestion by producing enzymes and bile that aid in breaking down food.

- **<u>Mouth and Esophagus:</u>**
    - Digestion begins in the mouth, where mechanical breakdown by chewing and chemical breakdown by saliva occur.
    - The esophagus is a muscular tube that transports food from the mouth to the stomach through peristaltic movements.

- **<u>Stomach:</u>**
    - The stomach is a hollow organ where food is mixed with gastric juices, including hydrochloric acid and digestive enzymes. This combination turns food into a semi-liquid substance called chyme.
    - The acidic environment in the stomach not only aids in breaking down food but also kills harmful bacteria and pathogens.

- **<u>Small Intestine:</u>**
    - The small intestine is the primary site for digestion and absorption of nutrients. It has three segments: the duodenum, jejunum, and ileum.
    - Enzymes from the pancreas and bile from the liver further digest food in the duodenum. The jejunum and ileum are mainly responsible for nutrient absorption.

- **<u>Large Intestine (Colon):</u>**
  - The large intestine absorbs water and electrolytes from indigestible food matter and forms solid waste (feces).
  - It also houses a vast array of gut bacteria that play a crucial role in fermenting undigested carbohydrates and synthesizing certain vitamins.

- **<u>Rectum and Anus:</u>**
  - The rectum stores feces until they are expelled from the body through the anus during defecation.

II.   <u>Importance of Digestive Health:</u>

Maintaining a healthy digestive system is vital for overall well-being. Here are several reasons why digestive health is crucial:

- **<u>Nutrient Absorption:</u>**
  - Efficient digestion ensures that the body absorbs essential nutrients, vitamins, and minerals from food, which are necessary for energy production, growth, and cellular repair.

- **<u>Immune Function:</u>**
  - The gut is home to a significant portion of the body's immune system. A healthy gut flora (microbiome) helps protect against pathogens and supports immune responses.

- **<u>Mental Health:</u>**
  - The gut-brain axis refers to the bidirectional communication between the gut and the brain. A healthy gut can positively influence mood and cognitive functions, reducing the risk of mental health issues such as anxiety and depression.

- **<u>Chronic Disease Prevention:</u>**
  - Proper digestive function and a balanced gut microbiome are associated with a lower risk of chronic diseases such as inflammatory bowel disease (IBD), irritable bowel syndrome (IBS), and metabolic disorders like obesity and diabetes.

III.   <u>Common Digestive Disorders:</u>

Digestive disorders can significantly impact quality of life. Here are some common conditions:

- **<u>Irritable Bowel Syndrome (IBS):</u>**
  - IBS is a functional gastrointestinal disorder characterized by symptoms such as abdominal pain, bloating, and altered bowel habits (constipation, diarrhea, or both).
  - The exact cause of IBS is unknown, but factors like stress, diet, and gut microbiome imbalances are believed to play a role.

- **<u>Inflammatory Bowel Disease (IBD):</u>**
  - IBD includes chronic inflammatory conditions of the digestive tract, primarily Crohn's disease and ulcerative colitis.
  - These conditions can cause severe symptoms such as abdominal pain, diarrhea, weight loss, and fatigue, and they often require long-term management.

- **<u>Gastroesophageal Reflux Disease (GERD):</u>**
  - GERD occurs when stomach acid frequently flows back into the esophagus, leading to symptoms such as heartburn, chest pain, and difficulty swallowing.
  - Lifestyle factors, diet, and obesity are common contributing factors to GERD.

- **<u>Celiac Disease:</u>**
  - Celiac disease is an autoimmune disorder where ingestion of gluten leads to damage in the small intestine.
  - Symptoms include diarrhea, bloating, fatigue, and malabsorption of nutrients. Strict adherence to a gluten-free diet is necessary for management.

- **<u>Diverticulitis:</u>**
  - Diverticulitis occurs when small, bulging pouches (diverticula) in the digestive tract become inflamed or infected.
  - It can cause severe abdominal pain, fever, and changes in bowel habits. A high-fiber diet may help prevent diverticulitis.

- **<u>Constipation and Diarrhea:</u>**
  - Constipation is characterized by infrequent or difficult bowel movements, often caused by a low-fiber diet, dehydration, or lack of physical activity.
  - Diarrhea involves frequent, loose, or watery stools and can be caused by infections, food intolerances, or chronic digestive conditions.

- **<u>Importance of Early Detection and Management:</u>**

  Early detection and effective management of digestive disorders are crucial for preventing complications and improving quality of life. Here are key strategies:

- **<u>Regular Medical Check-Ups:</u>**
  - Routine medical examinations can help detect digestive disorders early, allowing for timely intervention and management.

- **Dietary Modifications:**
  - Adjusting the diet to include fiber-rich foods, probiotics, and other gut-friendly nutrients can alleviate symptoms and promote digestive health.

- **Stress Management:**
  - Stress can exacerbate digestive symptoms. Techniques such as mindfulness, meditation, and exercise can help manage stress levels.

- **Hydration:**
  - Adequate water intake is essential for maintaining digestive function and preventing conditions like constipation.

- **Medication and Supplements:**
  - In some cases, medications and dietary supplements (e.g., probiotics, digestive enzymes) may be necessary to manage symptoms and support digestive health.

Conclusion:

Understanding the digestive system and its functions is the first step toward maintaining optimal digestive health. Recognizing the importance of a balanced diet, regular exercise, stress management, and early detection of digestive disorders can significantly improve overall health and well-being. As we continue through this book, we will explore in-depth strategies and dietary therapies to manage and prevent common digestive issues, promoting a healthier and more comfortable life.

Chapter 2
Understanding the Gut Microbiome

I.   <u>Role of the Microbiome in Digestion:</u>

The human gut is a bustling ecosystem teeming with trillions of microorganisms, collectively known as the gut microbiome. This complex community includes bacteria, viruses, fungi, and other microbes that play a pivotal role in digestion and overall health. These microorganisms assist in breaking down complex carbohydrates, proteins, and fats that our bodies cannot digest on their own. By producing enzymes, the microbiome helps in the digestion of dietary fibers, leading to the absorption of essential nutrients, vitamins, and minerals. Moreover, these microorganisms synthesize short-chain fatty acids (SCFAs) like butyrate, propionate, and acetate, which serve as vital energy sources for the cells lining the colon and help maintain the integrity of the gut barrier.

II.   <u>Factors Affecting Gut Health:</u>

Several factors influence the composition and health of the gut microbiome:

1. Diet:

Diet is the most significant determinant of microbiome composition. Diets rich in fiber from fruits, vegetables, and whole grains promote a diverse and healthy microbiome, whereas high-fat, high-sugar diets can lead to a less diverse microbiome associated with inflammation and metabolic disorders.

2. Antibiotics and Medications:

Antibiotics, while essential for fighting infections, can disrupt the balance of the gut microbiome by killing beneficial bacteria. Other medications, such as proton pump inhibitors and nonsteroidal anti-inflammatory drugs (NSAIDs), can also impact gut health.

3. Lifestyle Factors:

Stress, lack of sleep, and sedentary behavior negatively affect the gut microbiome. Chronic stress, for example, has been linked to changes in gut bacteria composition and increased gut permeability.

4. Age:

The gut microbiome evolves over a person's life. It is highly dynamic in early life, stabilizes in adulthood, and changes again in old age, often becoming less diverse.

5. Environmental Exposures:

Factors such as pollution, toxins, and household cleaning products can influence the microbiome's composition and functionality.

III.   <u>Probiotics and Prebiotics:</u>

To maintain or restore a healthy gut microbiome, probiotics and prebiotics can be particularly beneficial.

1. Probiotics:

Probiotics are live microorganisms that, when consumed in adequate amounts, confer health benefits on the host. They are found in fermented foods like yogurt, kefir, sauerkraut, kimchi, and kombucha, as well as in dietary supplements. Probiotics can help replenish beneficial bacteria in the gut, enhance immune function, and improve digestion.

2. Prebiotics:

Prebiotics are non-digestible food components that promote the growth and activity of beneficial bacteria in the gut. They are found in high-fiber foods such as garlic, onions, leeks, asparagus, bananas, and whole grains. Prebiotics serve as food for probiotics, supporting their growth and activity.

- ### **Interaction Between Probiotics and Prebiotics:**

When combined, probiotics and prebiotics create a synergistic relationship known as Synbiotics. This combination can more effectively support the gut microbiome by ensuring that the beneficial bacteria (probiotics) are well-nourished (by prebiotics) and can thrive.

- ### **Optimizing Gut Health Through Diet:**

1. Eat a Diverse Range of Foods:

A diverse diet leads to a diverse microbiome, which is associated with better health. Incorporating a wide variety of fruits, vegetables, legumes, and whole grains promotes a robust microbiome.

2. Include Fermented Foods:

Foods like yogurt, kefir, sauerkraut, kimchi, and kombucha are rich in probiotics and help maintain a healthy balance of gut bacteria.

3. Increase Fiber Intake:

Consuming foods high in dietary fiber, such as beans, lentils, oats, and fruits, supports the growth of beneficial bacteria in the gut.

4. Limit Processed Foods and Sugars:

Diets high in processed foods and sugars can negatively impact the gut microbiome by promoting the growth of harmful bacteria.

5. Stay Hydrated:

Adequate hydration supports digestion and helps maintain the mucosal lining of the intestines, promoting a healthy gut environment.

- ## <u>Strategies for Maintaining Gut Health:</u>

1. Regular Physical Activity:

Exercise is known to enhance gut health by increasing microbial diversity. Regular physical activity can also reduce the risk of developing digestive issues such as constipation.

2. Stress Management:

Chronic stress negatively impacts gut health. Techniques such as meditation, yoga, and deep-breathing exercises can help manage stress levels, thereby supporting a healthy gut microbiome.

3. Adequate Sleep:

Quality sleep is crucial for overall health, including gut health. Poor sleep can disrupt the balance of the gut microbiome, leading to various health issues.

4. Avoid Unnecessary Antibiotics:

Antibiotics should be used only when necessary, as they can significantly disrupt the gut microbiome. Always consult a healthcare professional before starting an antibiotic course.

- ### The Future of Gut Health Research:

Research on the gut microbiome is rapidly evolving, with new discoveries highlighting its importance in various aspects of health beyond digestion, including mental health, immune function, and chronic disease prevention. Advances in microbiome research could lead to novel therapies and personalized nutrition plans tailored to individual microbiome profiles, offering more effective ways to maintain and improve health.

- ### Case Studies and Success Stories:

1. Case Study: Sarah's IBS Journey:

Sarah, a 32-year-old woman suffering from irritable bowel syndrome (IBS), experienced significant relief after incorporating a diet rich in prebiotics and probiotics. By including more fermented foods and high-fiber vegetables, she noticed a reduction in bloating and abdominal pain within a few months.

2. Case Study: John's Recovery from Antibiotic Use:

John, who had to take a prolonged course of antibiotics for a bacterial infection, suffered from digestive issues post-treatment. By gradually introducing probiotics and prebiotics into his diet, he was able to restore his gut flora and improve his digestion.

3. Case Study: Emma's Fight Against Chronic Stress:

Emma, a high-stress executive, faced severe digestive problems linked to her lifestyle. Incorporating stress management techniques like yoga and mindfulness, along with a balanced diet rich in prebiotics and probiotics, helped her regain gut health and overall well-being.

Conclusion:

Understanding the gut microbiome and its profound impact on digestion and overall health is essential for anyone looking to optimize their digestive health. By focusing on a diverse, fiber-rich diet, incorporating probiotics and prebiotics, and being mindful of lifestyle factors, individuals can foster a thriving gut microbiome that supports not only digestive health but overall well-being. This knowledge empowers us to make informed choices that nurture our internal ecosystems and, by extension, our health and vitality.

Chapter 3
Dietary Interventions
for Common Digestive Disorders

I. Irritable Bowel Syndrome (IBS):

Irritable Bowel Syndrome (IBS) is a common functional gastrointestinal disorder characterized by symptoms such as abdominal pain, bloating, and altered bowel habits, including diarrhea, constipation, or both. While the exact cause of IBS is unknown, dietary interventions can significantly help manage symptoms.

• Low FODMAP Diet:

The Low FODMAP diet is a well-researched approach for managing IBS symptoms. It involves reducing the intake of certain types of carbohydrates that are poorly absorbed in the small intestine and easily fermented by gut bacteria, leading to symptoms.

- **Phase 1:** Elimination: During this initial phase, all high FODMAP foods are eliminated from the diet for 4-6 weeks. High FODMAP foods include certain fruits (like apples, pears), vegetables (such as onions, garlic), legumes, dairy products, wheat, and artificial sweeteners.
- **Phase 2:** Reintroduction: Foods are gradually reintroduced one at a time to identify which types trigger symptoms. Each food is tested for three days, starting with a small amount and increasing it if tolerated.
- **Phase 3:** Personalization: Based on the reintroduction results, a personalized eating plan is developed. This phase includes a mix of low and high FODMAP foods that the individual can tolerate without experiencing symptoms.

- **Fiber Intake:**

Balancing fiber intake is critical for managing IBS. Soluble fiber, which dissolves in water to form a gel-like substance, can help ease IBS symptoms. Sources of soluble fiber include oats, barley, carrots, and apples. Insoluble fiber, which does not dissolve in water, may exacerbate symptoms for some people and is found in whole grains and vegetables. A gradual increase in fiber intake, along with adequate hydration, is recommended to avoid exacerbating symptoms.

- **Probiotics:**

Probiotics are live microorganisms that can provide health benefits when consumed in adequate amounts. Certain probiotic strains, such as Bifidobacterium and Lactobacillus, have been shown to alleviate IBS symptoms by improving the balance of gut bacteria, reducing inflammation, and enhancing gut barrier function. Fermented foods like yogurt, kefir, sauerkraut, and kimchi are good sources of probiotics.

II.   Inflammatory Bowel Disease (IBD):

Inflammatory Bowel Disease (IBD), which includes Crohn's disease and ulcerative colitis, involves chronic inflammation of the digestive tract. While diet alone cannot cure IBD, it can significantly influence the severity and frequency of symptoms.

- **Specific Carbohydrate Diet (SCD):**

The Specific Carbohydrate Diet (SCD) restricts complex carbohydrates and focuses on simple, easily digestible foods to reduce inflammation and bacterial overgrowth.

- **Allowed Foods:** The diet includes meat, fish, eggs, nuts, fruits, and non-starchy vegetables. These foods are less likely to ferment in the gut and cause symptoms.
- **Avoided Foods:** Grains, starchy vegetables, processed foods, and certain dairy products are excluded from the diet, as they can contribute to inflammation and bacterial imbalance.

- **<u>Anti-inflammatory Diet:</u>**

An anti-inflammatory diet includes foods that help reduce inflammation in the body. These foods are rich in omega-3 fatty acids, antioxidants, and anti-inflammatory compounds.

- **Omega-3 Fatty Acids:** Found in fatty fish like salmon, mackerel, and sardines, as well as in flaxseeds and chia seeds, omega-3s help reduce inflammation.
- **Antioxidants:** Berries, leafy greens, and other colorful fruits and vegetables are rich in antioxidants, which help protect cells from damage.
- **Anti-inflammatory Compounds:** Foods like turmeric, ginger, and green tea contain natural anti-inflammatory compounds that can help manage IBD symptoms.

- **<u>Enteral Nutrition:</u>**

Enteral nutrition involves using a liquid diet to provide essential nutrients while giving the gut time to heal. This approach is especially useful during flare-ups. There are two main types of enteral nutrition:

- **Exclusive Enteral Nutrition (EEN):** Involves consuming only a liquid formula for a period of time, typically 6-8 weeks. This approach can induce remission in children and some adults with IBD.

- **Partial Enteral Nutrition (PEN):** Combines a liquid formula with regular food. This approach can help maintain remission and provide nutritional support.

III. Gastroesophageal Reflux Disease (GERD):

Gastroesophageal Reflux Disease (GERD) occurs when stomach acid frequently flows back into the esophagus, causing irritation and symptoms such as heartburn and acid reflux.

• Trigger Foods:

Identifying and avoiding trigger foods can help manage GERD symptoms. Common triggers include:

- **Spicy Foods:** Can irritate the esophagus and worsen reflux symptoms.
- **Fatty Foods:** Slow down digestion and increase the risk of reflux by relaxing the lower esophageal sphincter (LES).
- **Citrus Fruits:** Increase stomach acidity, which can exacerbate symptoms.
- **Caffeine and Alcohol:** Relax the LES, allowing stomach acid to flow back into the esophagus.

• Meal Timing and Portion Control:

Eating smaller, more frequent meals rather than large meals can help prevent reflux. Additionally, avoiding meals close to bedtime (at least 3 hours before lying down) can reduce nighttime symptoms.

• Dietary Modifications:
- Increase Fiber Intake: High-fiber foods like fruits, vegetables, and whole grains can help improve digestion and reduce reflux.

- Stay Hydrated: Drinking plenty of water helps neutralize stomach acid and aids digestion.
- Chewing Gum: Chewing sugar-free gum after meals can increase saliva production, which neutralizes acid and reduces symptoms.

- **<u>Integrative Approaches:</u>**

Combining dietary interventions with lifestyle modifications can enhance the management of digestive disorders. Here are some integrative strategies:

- **<u>Mind-Body Techniques:</u>**

Stress management is crucial, as stress can exacerbate digestive symptoms. Techniques such as mindfulness meditation, yoga, and cognitive-behavioral therapy (CBT) can help manage stress levels and support gut health.

- **<u>Regular Physical Activity:</u>**

Exercise promotes healthy digestion and can help alleviate symptoms of IBS, IBD, and GERD. Aim for at least 30 minutes of moderate exercise most days of the week. Activities like walking, cycling, and swimming are particularly beneficial.

- **<u>Adequate Sleep:</u>**

Poor sleep can worsen digestive symptoms. Establish a regular sleep schedule and create a relaxing bedtime routine to improve sleep quality. Avoiding caffeine and heavy meals before bedtime can also help.

- **Case Studies and Success Stories:**

1. Case Study: Mark's IBS Management with Low FODMAP Diet:

Mark, a 28-year-old accountant, suffered from severe IBS symptoms, including abdominal pain and bloating. After adopting a Low FODMAP diet and identifying his specific triggers, Mark experienced significant relief. He found that foods like garlic and onions were major triggers, and by avoiding them, he could manage his symptoms effectively. Regular consultations with a dietitian helped him maintain a balanced and symptom-free diet.

2. Case Study: Lisa's Journey with IBD and Anti-inflammatory Diet:

Lisa, a 35-year-old teacher, was diagnosed with Crohn's disease. By incorporating anti-inflammatory foods such as salmon, blueberries, and turmeric into her diet, she managed to keep her symptoms under control. During flare-ups, she used exclusive enteral nutrition to allow her gut to heal. Additionally, she practiced yoga and mindfulness, which helped her manage stress and improve her overall well-being.

3. Case Study: John's GERD Relief through Dietary Modifications:

John, a 45-year-old engineer, struggled with chronic heartburn and acid reflux. By eliminating trigger foods such as spicy dishes, fatty meals, and citrus fruits from his diet, he significantly reduced his GERD symptoms. John also made a habit of eating smaller meals and avoiding food close to bedtime. Chewing gum after meals provided additional relief by increasing saliva production and neutralizing stomach acid.

Conclusion:

Dietary interventions are a powerful tool in managing common digestive disorders like IBS, IBD, and GERD. By understanding the specific dietary needs and triggers for each condition, individuals can make informed choices that significantly improve their quality of life. Combining dietary changes with lifestyle modifications, such as stress management, regular exercise, and adequate sleep, further enhances digestive health and overall well-being. These strategies empower individuals to take control of their digestive health, leading to a more balanced and healthy life.

Chapter 4
Elimination Diets and Food Sensitivities

I. **Identifying Food Intolerances:**

Food intolerances, unlike food allergies, do not involve the immune system but can still cause significant discomfort and digestive issues. Common symptoms include bloating, gas, diarrhea, constipation, abdominal pain, and headaches. Identifying food intolerances can be challenging because symptoms often appear hours or even days after consuming the offending food, making it difficult to pinpoint the cause.

- **Common Food Intolerances:**
  1. **Lactose Intolerance:** Inability to digest lactose, the sugar found in milk and dairy products, due to a deficiency in the enzyme lactase. Symptoms include bloating, diarrhea, and abdominal cramps after consuming dairy.
  2. **Gluten Sensitivity:** Adverse reactions to gluten, a protein found in wheat, barley, and rye. Symptoms are similar to those of celiac disease but without the autoimmune response.
  3. **Fructose Malabsorption:** Difficulty absorbing fructose, a sugar found in fruits, honey, and some vegetables. Symptoms include bloating, gas, and diarrhea.
  4. **Histamine Intolerance:** Problems processing histamine, a compound found in aged cheeses, cured meats, and fermented foods. Symptoms can include headaches, hives, and digestive issues.
  5. **Sulfite Sensitivity:** Reactions to sulfites, preservatives found in wine, dried fruits, and some processed foods. Symptoms can range from mild headaches to severe asthma attacks.

II.   <u>Implementing an Elimination Diet:</u>

An elimination diet is a structured approach to identify food intolerances by removing suspected foods from the diet and then gradually reintroducing them while monitoring symptoms. This method helps to identify which foods are causing adverse reactions.

- ## <u>Steps for an Elimination Diet:</u>

1. Preparation:

- Keep a Food Diary: Record all foods and drinks consumed, along with any symptoms experienced, to identify patterns and potential triggers.
- Consult a Healthcare Professional: Work with a dietitian or healthcare provider to ensure nutritional needs are met during the elimination process. They can also help plan the diet and monitor for any nutritional deficiencies.

2. Elimination Phase (2-6 weeks):

- Remove All Suspected Trigger Foods: Eliminate all common allergens and irritants such as dairy, gluten, soy, eggs, nuts, shellfish, and processed foods. This phase requires strict adherence to ensure accurate results.
- Focus on Simple, Whole Foods: Eat a diet consisting of fruits, vegetables, lean meats, and gluten-free grains. Ensure the foods consumed are not processed or contain any hidden ingredients that could trigger symptoms.

3. Reintroduction Phase:

- Gradually Reintroduce Foods: Reintroduce one food at a time every 3-5 days, starting with a small amount and increasing the portion if no symptoms occur. This helps to clearly identify which foods are causing issues.

- Monitor and Record Symptoms: Keep a detailed record of any reactions to each reintroduced food. Symptoms may take hours or days to appear, so careful monitoring is essential.
- Identify Triggers: If symptoms return after reintroducing a specific food, it is likely a trigger and should be avoided.

4. Maintenance Phase:

- Develop a Long-term Eating Plan: Based on the reintroduction results, create a sustainable diet that avoids identified trigger foods while ensuring a balanced and nutritious intake. This plan should be tailored to individual needs and preferences.
- Regular Review and Adjustments: Periodically review and adjust the diet as needed. Food sensitivities can change over time, and new intolerances may develop.

- <u>**Common Challenges and Solutions:**</u>
1. **Nutrient Deficiencies:** Eliminating entire food groups can lead to nutrient deficiencies. Ensure a well-rounded diet by incorporating alternative sources of essential nutrients. For example, if dairy is eliminated, ensure adequate calcium and vitamin D from other sources like leafy greens, fortified plant-based milks, and supplements if necessary.
   - **Solution:** Work with a dietitian to identify nutrient gaps and find suitable food substitutes or supplements.

2. **Social and Emotional Impact:** Adhering to an elimination diet can be socially challenging and emotionally taxing. Planning ahead, bringing safe foods to social gatherings, and seeking support from friends, family, or support groups can help.

- **Solution:** Communicate your dietary needs with friends and family, plan meals in advance, and find a support network for emotional encouragement.

3. **Hidden Ingredients:** Many processed foods contain hidden ingredients that can trigger symptoms. Reading food labels carefully and cooking meals from scratch can minimize exposure to hidden triggers.
   - **Solution:** Learn to read food labels, avoid processed foods, and prepare meals at home using fresh, whole ingredients.

III.   Case Studies and Success Stories:

1. Case Study: Emma's Journey with Lactose Intolerance:

Emma, a 25-year-old student, experienced frequent bloating and diarrhea. By keeping a food diary, she noticed her symptoms worsened after consuming dairy products. Under the guidance of a dietitian, Emma eliminated dairy from her diet and saw significant improvement. She reintroduced dairy in small amounts to confirm her intolerance and now uses lactose-free products and calcium-fortified alternatives. Her symptoms have greatly improved, and she feels more energetic and less bloated.

2. Case Study: Mike's Struggle with Gluten Sensitivity:

Mike, a 40-year-old graphic designer, suffered from chronic fatigue and digestive issues. Despite testing negative for celiac disease, he decided to try a gluten-free elimination diet. After removing gluten, his symptoms dramatically improved. Through careful reintroduction, Mike confirmed his sensitivity and now follows a gluten-free diet, enjoying better energy levels and digestive health. He has found creative ways to enjoy his favorite foods using gluten-free alternatives.

3. Case Study: Sarah's Discovery of Histamine Intolerance:

Sarah, a 30-year-old marketing manager, experienced headaches, rashes, and digestive problems. Suspecting a histamine intolerance, she eliminated high-histamine foods like aged cheese, cured meats, and fermented foods. Her symptoms improved significantly, and through careful reintroduction, she identified her triggers. Sarah now manages her condition by limiting high-histamine foods and using antihistamines when needed. She has also discovered new recipes and foods that fit within her dietary restrictions, enhancing her overall health and well-being.

- ## Success Stories:

1. John's Triumph over Fructose Malabsorption:

John, a 35-year-old engineer, dealt with persistent bloating and diarrhea. After tracking his diet, he noticed symptoms flared after consuming fruits high in fructose. An elimination diet confirmed his fructose malabsorption. John now follows a low-fructose diet and enjoys significant relief from his symptoms. He has also learned to enjoy a variety of fruits and vegetables that are low in fructose, maintaining a balanced and nutritious diet.

2. Laura's Battle with Sulfite Sensitivity:

Laura, a 28-year-old artist, experienced frequent asthma attacks and digestive issues. Suspecting sulfite sensitivity, she eliminated foods and drinks high in sulfites, such as wine and dried fruits. Her symptoms improved, and through reintroduction, she confirmed her sensitivity. Laura now avoids sulfites and uses natural, preservative-free foods to maintain her health. She has also found ways to enjoy social gatherings and dining out without compromising her health.

Conclusion:

Elimination diets are a powerful tool for identifying and managing food intolerances. By systematically removing and reintroducing foods, individuals can pinpoint specific triggers and tailor their diets to avoid discomfort and digestive issues. While the process can be challenging, the rewards of improved health and well-being are well worth the effort. With careful planning, support, and guidance from healthcare professionals, individuals can navigate the complexities of food intolerances and enjoy a balanced, symptom-free diet.

Elimination diets not only help in identifying intolerances but also in understanding one's body and its unique needs. This knowledge empowers individuals to make informed dietary choices, leading to better digestive health and overall quality of life.

Chapter 5
Fiber: The Unsung Hero of Digestive Health

I. Types of Dietary Fiber:

Dietary fiber, found in plant-based foods, is crucial for maintaining digestive health. Fiber is classified into two main types: soluble fiber and insoluble fiber. Each type has unique properties and offers specific benefits to the digestive system.

- ### Soluble Fiber:

Soluble fiber dissolves in water to form a gel-like substance in the gut. This type of fiber slows digestion, helping to regulate blood sugar levels and lower cholesterol.

- **Sources:** Oats, barley, nuts, seeds, beans, lentils, peas, apples, oranges, carrots, and psyllium.

Benefits:

- **Regulates Blood Sugar:** By slowing digestion, soluble fiber helps prevent spikes in blood sugar levels, making it beneficial for individuals with diabetes.
- **Lowers Cholesterol:** Soluble fiber can bind to cholesterol in the digestive system, preventing its absorption and helping to lower overall cholesterol levels.
- **Supports Gut Health:** Soluble fiber serves as a food source for beneficial gut bacteria, promoting a healthy microbiome and the production of short-chain fatty acids that nourish colon cells.

- ### Insoluble Fiber:

Insoluble fiber does not dissolve in water and adds bulk to the stool, helping food pass more quickly through the stomach and intestines.

- **Sources:** Whole grains (such as whole wheat, brown rice, and oats), wheat bran, vegetables like cauliflower, green beans, and potatoes, nuts, and seeds.

Benefits:

- **Promotes Regularity:** By adding bulk to the stool, insoluble fiber helps to prevent constipation and promote regular bowel movements.
- **Maintains Digestive Health:** Insoluble fiber helps maintain an optimal pH in the intestines, which can prevent harmful bacteria from proliferating.
- **Prevents Digestive Disorders:** Regular consumption of insoluble fiber can reduce the risk of developing hemorrhoids and diverticulitis by ensuring smooth bowel movements.

II.   Benefits of Fiber for Digestion:

Dietary fiber provides numerous benefits for the digestive system, contributing to overall health and well-being.

• Promotes Regularity:

Fiber increases stool bulk and helps it move more quickly through the digestive tract, preventing constipation and promoting regular bowel movements. Regularity reduces the risk of developing hemorrhoids and diverticular disease. Insoluble fiber is particularly effective in this regard, ensuring that waste moves efficiently through the colon.

• Supports a Healthy Gut Microbiome:

Fiber, especially soluble fiber, acts as a prebiotic, feeding beneficial gut bacteria. A healthy gut microbiome is essential for effective digestion, nutrient absorption, and a strong immune system. Beneficial bacteria ferment soluble fiber, producing short-chain fatty acids like butyrate, which provide energy to colon cells and reduce inflammation.

- **<u>Manages Blood Sugar Levels:</u>**

Soluble fiber slows the absorption of sugar, helping to regulate blood sugar levels. This is particularly beneficial for individuals with diabetes or those at risk of developing the condition. By slowing the digestive process, fiber helps prevent the rapid rise and fall of blood sugar levels, providing more stable energy levels.

- **<u>Lowers Cholesterol Levels:</u>**

Soluble fiber binds to cholesterol in the digestive system, preventing its absorption into the bloodstream. This can help lower overall cholesterol levels and reduce the risk of heart disease. By reducing the amount of cholesterol that enters the bloodstream, fiber contributes to cardiovascular health.

- **<u>Helps with Weight Management:</u>**

High-fiber foods are more filling, which can help control appetite and reduce overall calorie intake. This is beneficial for weight management and preventing obesity-related digestive issues. Fiber-rich foods take longer to chew and digest, which helps individuals feel full longer and prevents overeating.

III. <u>High-Fiber Meal Plans and Recipes:</u>

Incorporating more fiber into your diet can be delicious and easy with a variety of high-fiber meal plans and recipes. A balanced approach includes both soluble and insoluble fiber from diverse sources.

- **<u>Sample High-Fiber Meal Plan:</u>**

Breakfast:

- **Oatmeal with Berries and Nuts:** Cooked oats topped with fresh berries, a tablespoon of chia seeds, and a handful of almonds. Oats provide soluble fiber, while berries and nuts add both soluble and insoluble fiber.
- **Smoothie:** Blend spinach, banana, apple, and a tablespoon of flaxseeds with almond milk. This smoothie is packed with fiber from fruits, greens, and seeds.

Lunch:

Quinoa Salad: Quinoa mixed with black beans, corn, diced tomatoes, avocado, and a lime-cilantro dressing. Quinoa and black beans are excellent sources of fiber, while vegetables add bulk and nutrients.

Vegetable Soup: A hearty soup with lentils, carrots, celery, spinach, and tomatoes. Lentils are rich in fiber, and the variety of vegetables adds additional fiber and nutrients.

Dinner:

Grilled Chicken with Brown Rice and Broccoli: Grilled chicken breast served with a side of brown rice and steamed broccoli. Brown rice and broccoli provide insoluble fiber, aiding digestion.

Stir-Fried Vegetables: A mix of bell peppers, snap peas, carrots, and tofu stir-fried in olive oil with garlic and ginger. This dish combines the fiber from various vegetables and protein from tofu.

Snacks:

Fruit and Nut Mix: A handful of mixed nuts and dried apricots. Nuts and dried fruits are convenient, fiber-rich snacks.

Hummus with Carrot Sticks: Homemade or store-bought hummus served with fresh carrot sticks. Chickpeas in hummus are high in fiber, and carrots provide crunch and additional fiber.

- ## **High-Fiber Recipes:**

Lentil and Vegetable Stew:

- **Ingredients:** Lentils, carrots, celery, onions, tomatoes, spinach, garlic, vegetable broth, olive oil, salt, and pepper.
- **Instructions:**

  1. Sauté onions, garlic, carrots, and celery in olive oil until soft.

  2. Add lentils, tomatoes, and vegetable broth.

  3. Simmer until lentils are cooked through.

  4. Stir in spinach and cook until wilted.

  5. Season with salt and pepper to taste.

Berry Chia Pudding:

- **Ingredients:** Chia seeds, almond milk, vanilla extract, honey, mixed berries.
- **Instructions:**

  1. Mix chia seeds, almond milk, vanilla extract, and honey in a bowl.

  2. Refrigerate for at least 4 hours or overnight until the mixture thickens.

  3. Top with mixed berries before serving.

Quinoa and Black Bean Salad:

- **Ingredients:** Cooked quinoa, black beans, corn, red bell pepper, avocado, lime juice, cilantro, olive oil, salt, and pepper.
- **Instructions:**

  1. Mix cooked quinoa, black beans, corn, and diced red bell pepper in a large bowl.

  2. Add diced avocado, lime juice, chopped cilantro, and olive oil.

  3. Season with salt and pepper and toss to combine.

- **Tips for Increasing Fiber Intake:**
1. **Start Slow:** Gradually increase fiber intake to allow your digestive system to adjust and prevent gas and bloating. Sudden increases in fiber can cause discomfort, so it's best to introduce fiber slowly.
2. **Stay Hydrated:** Drink plenty of water to help fiber move smoothly through the digestive tract. Water helps soluble fiber form a gel-like consistency and assists insoluble fiber in adding bulk to stools.
3. **Incorporate Fiber-Rich Foods:** Add fruits, vegetables, whole grains, legumes, nuts, and seeds to every meal. These foods are naturally high in fiber and contribute to overall health.
4. **Choose Whole Foods:** Opt for whole fruits and vegetables rather than juices or processed foods. Whole foods retain their fiber content, while processing often removes fiber.
5. **Read Labels:** Look for high-fiber options when buying packaged foods. Foods labeled "whole grain" or "high fiber" are better choices for increasing fiber intake.

<u>Conclusion:</u>

Fiber is an essential component of a healthy diet, offering numerous benefits for digestive health. By understanding the different types of fiber and their roles, individuals can make informed dietary choices to improve their digestion, support a healthy gut microbiome, and enhance overall well-being. Incorporating a variety of high-fiber foods into daily meals can be both delicious and beneficial, leading to a healthier and more balanced lifestyle.

The importance of fiber cannot be overstated. It is a key factor in maintaining digestive health, managing weight, and preventing chronic diseases. By prioritizing fiber-rich foods and following practical tips for increasing fiber intake, individuals can experience significant improvements in their digestive health and overall quality of life.

Chapter 6
The Role of Hydration in Digestion

Water is a cornerstone of health, and its role in digestion is vital. From breaking down food to facilitating nutrient absorption and ensuring smooth passage through the intestines, hydration is key. This chapter explores the multifaceted importance of water and other fluids in maintaining digestive health, providing detailed insights and practical tips for optimal hydration.

I. <u>Importance of Water and Fluids:</u>

Water is essential for various bodily functions, and its role in the digestive system is particularly crucial. Hydration impacts every stage of the digestive process, from breaking down food to nutrient absorption and waste elimination.

- **Breaking Down Food:**
  - **Digestive Enzymes:** Water is necessary for the production and function of digestive enzymes. These enzymes break down food into smaller, absorbable molecules. Without sufficient water, enzyme activity is impaired, leading to incomplete digestion and reduced nutrient absorption.
  - **Saliva Production:** Saliva, which is mostly water, begins the digestive process by moistening food and initiating the breakdown of carbohydrates with the enzyme amylase. Saliva also helps in forming a food bolus, making it easier to swallow.
- **Transporting Nutrients:**
  - **Absorption:** Water facilitates the absorption of nutrients in the intestines. Nutrients need to be dissolved in water to pass through the intestinal lining into the bloodstream.
  - **Circulation:** Adequate hydration ensures efficient blood circulation, which is essential for transporting absorbed nutrients to various cells and tissues throughout the body.

- **Eliminating Waste:**
  - **Stool Formation:** Water helps to soften stool, making it easier to pass and preventing constipation. Dehydration can lead to hard, dry stools that are difficult to expel, causing discomfort and potential complications such as hemorrhoids.
  - **Kidney Function:** Water is crucial for kidney function. It helps filter waste products from the blood and excretes them through urine. Adequate hydration ensures that the kidneys can effectively remove toxins and maintain electrolyte balance.
- **Regulating Body Temperature:**
  - **Sweating:** Water helps regulate body temperature through sweating. Proper hydration ensures that the body can effectively cool itself, which is important for overall homeostasis and digestive function. When the body is overheated, it prioritizes cooling mechanisms over digestion, which can disrupt digestive processes.

II.   Hydration Tips for Optimal Digestion:

Ensuring adequate hydration is essential for maintaining digestive health. Here are some practical tips to help you stay hydrated and support your digestive system:

- **Drink Plenty of Water:**
  - **Daily Intake:** Aim to drink at least 8 glasses (about 2 liters) of water per day. This amount may vary depending on factors such as age, gender, activity level, and climate. Individual hydration needs can vary, so it's important to listen to your body.
  - **Consistency:** Sip water throughout the day rather than consuming large amounts at once. This helps maintain steady hydration levels and supports continuous digestive function.
- **Incorporate Hydrating Foods:**
  - **Fruits and Vegetables:** Foods with high water content, such as cucumbers, tomatoes, watermelon, strawberries, and oranges,

contribute to overall hydration. These foods also provide vitamins, minerals, and fiber, which support digestive health.

- **Soups and Broths:** Including soups and broths in your diet can also help increase your fluid intake. These can be particularly beneficial in colder weather when people may drink less water.

- **Limit Dehydrating Beverages:**
    - **Caffeine and Alcohol:** Both caffeine and alcohol can have diuretic effects, leading to increased urine output and potential dehydration. Consume these beverages in moderation and balance them with water intake. For example, for every cup of coffee or alcoholic drink, have a glass of water.
    - **Sugary Drinks:** Avoid sugary drinks like soda, which can contribute to dehydration and provide little nutritional benefit. Sugary beverages can also lead to weight gain and other health issues that can negatively impact digestion.

- **Monitor Hydration Levels:**
    - **Urine Color:** A simple way to gauge your hydration status is by observing the color of your urine. Light yellow or clear urine typically indicates good hydration, while dark yellow suggests you need more fluids. If your urine is consistently dark, it's a sign that you need to increase your water intake.
    - **Thirst Cues:** Pay attention to your body's signals. Thirst is a late indicator of dehydration, so try to drink water regularly before you feel thirsty. Other signs of dehydration include dry mouth, fatigue, and dizziness.

III. **Herbal Teas and Digestive Health:**

Herbal teas can be a beneficial addition to your hydration routine, offering both hydration and specific digestive benefits. Many herbal teas contain compounds that can soothe the digestive tract, reduce inflammation, and promote overall digestive health.

- **Peppermint Tea:**
    - **Digestive Aid:** Peppermint tea is known for its ability to relieve digestive issues such as bloating, gas, and indigestion. The menthol

in peppermint has antispasmodic properties that can relax the muscles of the gastrointestinal tract, alleviating discomfort.
- **Soothing Effect:** It also has a soothing effect on the stomach lining and can help alleviate symptoms of irritable bowel syndrome (IBS). Peppermint tea can be particularly helpful after a heavy meal.

- **Ginger Tea:**
  - **Nausea Relief:** Ginger tea is well-known for its ability to combat nausea and vomiting, making it an excellent choice for those with motion sickness or morning sickness. Ginger can also stimulate saliva, bile, and gastric juice production, which aids in digestion.
  - **Anti-Inflammatory:** Ginger contains anti-inflammatory compounds called gingerols that can help reduce inflammation in the digestive tract, promoting overall digestive health.

- **Chamomile Tea:**
  - **Calming Properties:** Chamomile tea has calming effects that can help reduce stress and anxiety, which are often linked to digestive issues. Its gentle sedative effects can promote relaxation and better digestion.
  - **Anti-Inflammatory:** It also has anti-inflammatory and antispasmodic properties that can help soothe the digestive tract and relieve cramps and spasms. Chamomile tea can be particularly beneficial for individuals with IBS or gastritis.

- **Fennel Tea:**
  - **Digestive Support:** Fennel tea can help relieve bloating, gas, and stomach cramps. It acts as a carminative, reducing gas formation and aiding in its expulsion. Fennel can also stimulate the production of gastric enzymes.
  - **Antimicrobial:** Fennel has antimicrobial properties that can help maintain a healthy balance of gut bacteria, promoting overall digestive health.

- **<u>Dandelion Tea:</u>**
  - **Liver Support:** Dandelion tea supports liver function, which is crucial for digestion and detoxification. A healthy liver ensures efficient bile production, which aids in the digestion of fats.
  - **Diuretic:** It acts as a mild diuretic, helping to flush out toxins and reduce water retention. Dandelion tea can also promote appetite and relieve digestive ailments such as constipation and indigestion.

Conclusion:

Hydration is a fundamental aspect of digestive health. Adequate water and fluid intake ensure that the digestive system functions smoothly, from breaking down food to absorbing nutrients and eliminating waste. Incorporating hydrating foods and herbal teas can further enhance your digestive health, providing specific benefits that support various aspects of digestion. By following these hydration tips and understanding the role of fluids in digestion, you can maintain optimal digestive health and overall well-being. Proper hydration is not just about drinking enough water; it's about supporting every aspect of the digestive process and ensuring that your body can efficiently process and utilize the nutrients you consume.

Chapter 7
Nutritional Strategies for Managing Constipation and Diarrhea

Constipation and diarrhea are two prevalent gastrointestinal issues that can significantly impact an individual's daily life and overall health. Managing these conditions effectively requires a thorough understanding of their causes and implementing targeted nutritional strategies. This chapter provides detailed insights into dietary causes and solutions for constipation and diarrhea, along with practical tips and meal suggestions to aid in their management.

I. <u>Dietary Causes and Solutions for Constipation:</u>

Constipation is often characterized by infrequent, difficult, or painful bowel movements. Understanding the dietary factors that contribute to constipation can help in crafting effective management strategies.

- **<u>Dietary Causes:</u>**

  ### 1. Low Fiber Intake:

  - **Explanation:** Fiber plays a crucial role in adding bulk to stool and promoting regular bowel movements. A diet lacking in fiber can lead to harder, drier stools that are difficult to pass.
  - **Sources:** Fiber-rich foods include fruits (such as apples, berries, and pears), vegetables (such as carrots, spinach, and broccoli), whole grains (such as oats, brown rice, and whole wheat), legumes (such as beans, lentils, and chickpeas), nuts, and seeds.

2. Inadequate Fluid Intake:

- **Explanation:** Proper hydration is essential for maintaining the softness of stool. Inadequate water intake can result in hard, dry stools that are challenging to pass.
- Sources: Drink plenty of water throughout the day. Hydrating foods like cucumbers, oranges, and strawberries can also contribute to fluid intake.

3. High Consumption of Processed Foods:

- **Explanation:** Processed foods are often low in fiber and high in fats and sugars, which can contribute to constipation by slowing down the digestive process.
- Sources: Processed foods include fast food, packaged snacks, sugary cereals, and ready-to-eat meals.

4. Sedentary Lifestyle:

- **Explanation:** Physical inactivity can reduce bowel motility, leading to constipation. Regular movement helps stimulate the digestive system and promote regular bowel movements.
- **Sources:** Incorporate activities like walking, jogging, cycling, and strength training into your daily routine.

- **<u>Nutritional Solutions:</u>**

  ### 1. Increase Fiber Intake:

- **Soluble Fiber:** Helps absorb water and form a gel-like substance that softens stool. Examples include oats, apples, and beans.
- **Insoluble Fiber:** Adds bulk to stool and aids its movement through the intestines. Sources include whole grains, nuts, and vegetables like cauliflower and zucchini.

2. Boost Fluid Intake:

- **Water:** Aim for at least 8 glasses of water daily to maintain proper hydration.
- **Hydrating Foods:** Include fruits and vegetables with high water content in your diet to enhance fluid intake.

3. Reduce Processed Foods:

- **Whole Foods:** Focus on whole, unprocessed foods such as fresh fruits, vegetables, and lean proteins to increase fiber and improve digestion.
- **Healthy Fats:** Opt for sources of healthy fats like avocados, nuts, and olive oil, and avoid excessive consumption of fried and greasy foods.

4. Regular Physical Activity:

- **Exercise Routine:** Engage in at least 30 minutes of moderate exercise most days of the week to enhance bowel function and alleviate constipation.

II.   Managing Diarrhea Through Diet:

Diarrhea is characterized by frequent, loose, or watery bowel movements and can be caused by various factors, including infections, food intolerances, and digestive disorders. Effective management involves dietary adjustments to alleviate symptoms and prevent dehydration.

- **Dietary Causes:**

  ### 1. Infections:

  - **Explanation:** Viral, bacterial, or parasitic infections can cause diarrhea by irritating the digestive tract and disrupting normal bowel function.
  - **Sources:** Contaminated food or water, poor hygiene, and certain medications.

  ### 2. Food Intolerances:

  - **Explanation:** Sensitivities to certain foods, such as lactose or gluten, can lead to diarrhea in susceptible individuals.
  - Sources: Dairy products, gluten-containing grains, and specific allergens.

  ### 3. High-Fat Foods:

  - **Explanation:** Consuming high-fat foods can exacerbate diarrhea, particularly in individuals with conditions like irritable bowel syndrome (IBS).
  - **Sources:** Fried foods, greasy meals, and rich desserts.

- **Nutritional Solutions:**

  ### 1. Follow the BRAT Diet:

  - **Bananas:** Provide essential nutrients and help to firm up stool.
  - Rice: Plain white rice is gentle on the stomach and helps to bind stool.
  - **Applesauce:** Contains pectin, which can help solidify stool.
  - Toast: Plain toast is easy to digest and absorbs excess fluids in the digestive tract.

2. Stay Hydrated:

- **Oral Rehydration Solutions:** Use solutions or electrolyte drinks to replace lost fluids and electrolytes.
- **Clear Broths:** These provide hydration and essential nutrients without aggravating the digestive system.

3. Avoid Trigger Foods:

- **High-Fat Foods:** Reduce intake of foods high in fats and oils that can aggravate diarrhea.
- **Dairy Products:** Avoid dairy if you are lactose intolerant or if it exacerbates symptoms.
- **Sugary and Caffeinated Beverages:** Limit intake of beverages that can increase bowel movements and contribute to dehydration.

4. Gradually Reintroduce Foods:

- **Small, Frequent Meals:** Eat smaller, more frequent meals to avoid overwhelming the digestive system.
- **Bland Foods:** Reintroduce bland foods such as boiled potatoes, plain chicken, and steamed vegetables.

- <u>**Practical Tips and Meal Suggestions for Diarrhea:**</u>
  - **Breakfast:** Begin with plain toast and a small serving of applesauce, along with a banana.
  - **Lunch:** Have a simple meal with plain white rice, boiled chicken, and steamed carrots.
  - **Dinner:** Choose bland foods like plain pasta with a small amount of olive oil and boiled potatoes.
  - **Snacks:** Opt for easy-to-digest snacks like plain crackers, a small serving of plain yogurt (if tolerated), or clear broth.

III. **<u>Practical Tips and Meal Suggestions:</u>**

- **Breakfast:** Start your day with a bowl of oatmeal topped with fresh berries and a tablespoon of chia seeds. This provides a high-fiber start to the day.
- **Lunch:** Enjoy a colorful salad with mixed greens, chickpeas, cherry tomatoes, cucumbers, and a whole-grain roll on the side.
- **Dinner:** Opt for grilled salmon with a side of quinoa and steamed broccoli. This meal is rich in fiber and essential nutrients.
- **Snacks:** Choose high-fiber snacks like apple slices with almond butter, a handful of nuts, or carrot sticks with hummus.

Conclusion:

Effectively managing constipation and diarrhea through diet requires a comprehensive understanding of the dietary causes and solutions for each condition. By increasing fiber intake, staying hydrated, and making appropriate food choices, individuals can alleviate symptoms of constipation and promote regular bowel movements. For diarrhea, following a bland diet, staying hydrated, and avoiding trigger foods are essential for symptom relief and recovery. Practical meal suggestions and tips ensure that dietary adjustments are straightforward and effective, supporting better digestive health and overall well-being.

Chapter 8
Integrating Fermented Foods into Your Diet

Fermented foods have been a staple in many cultures for centuries, celebrated for their unique flavors and potential health benefits. They play a crucial role in supporting gut health due to their rich probiotic content, which can aid in digestion and improve the balance of gut bacteria. This chapter explores the benefits of fermented foods, common types, their preparation, and delicious recipes to help you easily incorporate them into your diet.

I. <u>Benefits of Fermented Foods:</u>

1. Probiotics and Gut Health:

- Fermented foods are rich in probiotics, which are beneficial bacteria that support a healthy gut microbiome.
- These probiotics can help improve digestion, enhance nutrient absorption, and boost the immune system.
- Regular consumption of fermented foods can help maintain a healthy balance of gut bacteria, potentially alleviating symptoms of digestive disorders such as irritable bowel syndrome (IBS) and inflammatory bowel disease (IBD).

2. Enhanced Nutrient Absorption:

- Fermentation can increase the bioavailability of nutrients, making them easier for the body to absorb.
- For example, the fermentation process can break down phytic acid in grains and legumes, enhancing the absorption of minerals like iron and zinc.
- Vitamins, especially B vitamins and vitamin K, are also synthesized during fermentation, providing additional nutritional benefits.

3. Improved Digestion:

- Fermented foods can aid in the digestion of complex carbohydrates and proteins.
- The enzymes produced during fermentation can help break down these macronutrients, making them easier to digest and reducing the likelihood of digestive discomfort.
- Additionally, probiotics can enhance the gut lining's function, reducing permeability and protecting against toxins and pathogens.

4. Immune Support:

- A significant portion of the immune system is located in the gut.
- By promoting a healthy gut microbiome, fermented foods can help strengthen the immune response and protect against infections.
- The production of antimicrobial peptides during fermentation can also help inhibit the growth of harmful bacteria.

5. Detoxification:

- Fermented foods can help detoxify the body by binding to and neutralizing toxins and heavy metals.
- They also aid in the excretion of waste products, promoting regular bowel movements and reducing the load on the liver.

II.   __Common Fermented Foods and Their Preparation:__

1. Yogurt:

- Made by fermenting milk with bacterial cultures, yogurt is a versatile and delicious source of probiotics.
- **Preparation:** Heat milk to about 180°F (82°C) to kill any undesirable bacteria, then cool it to 110°F (43°C). Add a yogurt

starter culture or a few tablespoons of plain yogurt with live cultures. Incubate the mixture at a warm temperature (110°F/43°C) for 6-12 hours until it thickens.

2. Kefir:

- A fermented milk drink that is tangy and slightly effervescent, kefir contains a diverse array of probiotics.
- **Preparation:** Add kefir grains to milk and let it ferment at room temperature for 24-48 hours. Stir occasionally to ensure even fermentation. Strain out the grains and store the kefir in the refrigerator.

3. Sauerkraut:

- Fermented cabbage with a tangy flavor, sauerkraut is rich in probiotics and vitamins.
- **Preparation:** Finely shred cabbage and mix with salt (2% of the cabbage weight). Pack the cabbage tightly into a jar, ensuring it is submerged in its own juice. Cover the jar with a cloth and let it ferment at room temperature for 1-4 weeks, checking occasionally for mold or yeast growth.

4. Kimchi:

- A traditional Korean dish made from fermented vegetables, typically including cabbage and radishes, seasoned with garlic, ginger, and chili pepper.
- **Preparation:** Chop vegetables and mix with salt, letting them sit to draw out moisture. Add a paste made from garlic, ginger, chili flakes, and fish sauce. Pack the mixture tightly into a jar and let it ferment at room temperature for 3-7 days.

5. Kombucha:

- A fermented tea drink that is slightly fizzy and contains probiotics, antioxidants, and vitamins.
- **Preparation:** Brew tea (black or green) and sweeten it with sugar. Add a SCOBY (symbiotic culture of bacteria and yeast) to the cooled tea. Cover with a cloth and let it ferment at room temperature for 7-14 days. Remove the SCOBY and bottle the kombucha, allowing it to carbonate for a few more days if desired.

III. <u>Recipes Featuring Fermented Ingredients:</u>

1. Greek Yogurt Parfait:

- **Ingredients:** Greek yogurt, fresh berries, honey, granola.
- **Instructions:** Layer Greek yogurt with fresh berries, drizzle with honey, and top with granola for a nutritious and probiotic-rich breakfast or snack.

2. Kefir Smoothie:

- **Ingredients:** Kefir, frozen berries, banana, spinach, honey.
- **Instructions:** Blend kefir with frozen berries, banana, spinach, and a drizzle of honey for a refreshing and gut-friendly smoothie.

3. Sauerkraut Salad:

- **Ingredients:** Sauerkraut, chopped apples, shredded carrots, raisins, olive oil, lemon juice.
- **Instructions:** Mix sauerkraut with chopped apples, shredded carrots, and raisins. Dress with olive oil and lemon juice for a tangy and crunchy salad.

4. Kimchi Fried Rice:

- **Ingredients:** Cooked rice, kimchi, diced vegetables (carrots, peas, bell peppers), soy sauce, sesame oil, egg.
- **Instructions:** Sauté diced vegetables in sesame oil, add kimchi and cooked rice, and stir-fry with soy sauce. Push the rice to one side of the pan and scramble an egg in the empty space, then mix it all together.

5. Kombucha Mocktail:

- **Ingredients:** Kombucha, sparkling water, fresh fruit juice, mint leaves.
- **Instructions:** Mix kombucha with sparkling water and a splash of fresh fruit juice. Garnish with mint leaves for a refreshing and probiotic-rich mocktail.

- ## <u>Incorporating Fermented Foods into Your Diet:</u>

  ### 1. Start Slowly:

  - Introduce fermented foods gradually to allow your digestive system to adjust.
  - Start with small portions and increase as tolerated to avoid potential digestive discomfort.

  ### 2. Variety is Key:

  - Incorporate a variety of fermented foods to benefit from different strains of probiotics and a broader range of nutrients.
  - Rotate between yogurt, kefir, sauerkraut, kimchi, and kombucha to keep your diet interesting and balanced.

3. Pair with Meals:

- Add a spoonful of sauerkraut or kimchi to your meals as a condiment.
- Enjoy a glass of kefir with breakfast or a kombucha mocktail with lunch.

4. Experiment with Recipes:

- Try new recipes that incorporate fermented foods to discover new flavors and textures.
- Use fermented foods as ingredients in salads, smoothies, sandwiches, and more.

5. Educate and Explore:

- Learn about the different types of fermented foods available in various cuisines.
- Explore local markets and specialty stores for new and interesting fermented products.

Conclusion:

Integrating fermented foods into your diet can provide numerous health benefits, particularly for digestive health. These foods are rich in probiotics, which support a healthy gut microbiome, enhance nutrient absorption, and improve digestion. By understanding the benefits and learning how to prepare and incorporate a variety of fermented foods, you can enjoy their unique flavors and health advantages. Start slowly, experiment with different recipes, and make fermented foods a regular part of your diet to promote optimal gut health and overall well-being.

By adopting these nutritional strategies, individuals can proactively manage their digestive health, prevent recurrence of symptoms, and enhance their overall well-being. This chapter provides a comprehensive guide to understanding and integrating fermented foods, offering practical advice and meal suggestions to support long-term digestive health.

Chapter 9
Dietary Approaches to SIBO and Candida Overgrowth

Small Intestinal Bacterial Overgrowth (SIBO) and Candida overgrowth are two common yet often misunderstood conditions that can significantly impact digestive health. Proper dietary management is crucial in addressing these issues effectively. This chapter provides a comprehensive guide to understanding SIBO and Candida overgrowth, dietary protocols for managing these conditions, and real-life case studies that illustrate successful interventions.

I. Understanding SIBO and Candida Overgrowth:

- ### Small Intestinal Bacterial Overgrowth (SIBO):

Definition and Causes:

SIBO occurs when excessive bacteria proliferate in the small intestine, leading to symptoms such as bloating, abdominal pain, diarrhea, and malabsorption. Normal bacterial populations are typically confined to the large intestine, but in SIBO, these bacteria move into the small intestine, disrupting normal digestion.

Causes:

- **Motility Issues:** Conditions such as irritable bowel syndrome (IBS) and diabetes can impair the natural movement of the intestines, allowing bacteria to accumulate.
- **Structural Abnormalities:** Conditions like diverticulosis or previous abdominal surgeries can create areas where bacteria can thrive.
- **Low Stomach Acid:** Reduced stomach acid production can fail to kill off harmful bacteria, allowing them to reach and overpopulate the small intestine.

Symptoms:

Bloating and distension

Excessive gas and belching

Diarrhea or constipation

Abdominal pain and cramping

Nutrient deficiencies and unintended weight loss

- ## <u>Candida Overgrowth:</u>

  ### Definition and Causes:

  Candida is a type of yeast that naturally resides in the gastrointestinal tract. However, an overgrowth of Candida can lead to various health issues. This condition often results from an imbalance in gut flora, allowing Candida to proliferate uncontrollably.

Causes:

- **Antibiotic Use:** Broad-spectrum antibiotics can disrupt the balance of gut flora, allowing Candida to grow unchecked.
- **High Sugar Diet:** Excessive sugar intake can feed Candida, promoting its overgrowth.
- **Immune System Imbalance:** Conditions that weaken the immune system, such as diabetes or autoimmune diseases, can make individuals more susceptible to Candida overgrowth.

Symptoms:

Persistent fatigue

Recurring yeast infections

Digestive issues such as bloating, gas, and diarrhea

Oral thrush (white patches in the mouth)

Skin rashes and itching

II. <u>Dietary Protocols for Managing SIBO and Candida Overgrowth:</u>

- **<u>SIBO Dietary Protocols:</u>**

1. Low FODMAP Diet:

- **Overview:** The Low FODMAP diet involves reducing the intake of fermentable oligosaccharides, disaccharides, monosaccharides, and polyols (FODMAPs) which are known to feed bacteria and exacerbate SIBO symptoms.
- **Foods to Avoid:** Garlic, onions, apples, pears, wheat, and certain dairy products.
- **Foods to Include:** Lean proteins, low-FODMAP vegetables (e.g., spinach, carrots), and low-FODMAP fruits (e.g., bananas, berries).

2. Specific Carbohydrate Diet (SCD):

- **Overview:** The SCD eliminates complex carbohydrates and sugars to reduce bacterial fermentation and support gut healing.
- **Foods to Avoid:** Grains, processed foods, and sugars.
- **Foods to Include:** Fresh meats, fish, eggs, non-starchy vegetables, and nuts.

3. Elemental Diet:

- **Overview:** This involves consuming a liquid diet of pre-digested nutrients, allowing the gut to rest and heal while reducing bacterial load.
- **Products:** Elemental shakes that are nutritionally complete and easily absorbed.

4. Probiotics and Prebiotics:

- **Overview:** Probiotics can help restore a healthy balance of gut bacteria, while prebiotics can help support this balance.
- **Recommended Strains:** Lactobacillus and Bifidobacterium strains are often recommended for SIBO.

- **Candida Dietary Protocols:**

1. Candida Diet:

- **Overview:** The Candida diet focuses on eliminating foods that promote yeast growth and supporting the body's ability to fight off Candida.
- **Foods to Avoid:** Sugar, refined grains, yeast-containing foods, and high-carb fruits.
- **Foods to Include:** Non-starchy vegetables, lean proteins, coconut oil, and anti-fungal foods such as garlic and ginger.

2. Anti-Fungal Diet:

- **Overview:** Incorporates foods and supplements that have natural anti-fungal properties to combat Candida overgrowth.
- **Foods to Include:** Garlic, coconut oil, oregano oil, and apple cider vinegar.

3. Reintroducing Foods:

- **Overview:** Once symptoms are under control, gradually reintroduce foods to determine which ones trigger symptoms.
- **Approach:** Monitor symptoms closely and adjust dietary choices based on individual tolerance.

III. Real-Life Case Studies:

Case Study 1: Managing SIBO with the Low FODMAP Diet:

- **Patient Background:** Sarah, a 35-year-old woman, struggled with bloating and abdominal pain. After undergoing a breath test, she was diagnosed with SIBO.
- **Dietary Intervention:** Sarah adopted the Low FODMAP diet, avoiding high-FODMAP foods and focusing on low-FODMAP options.
- **Outcome:** After three months, Sarah experienced a significant reduction in symptoms, including decreased bloating and pain. She reported improved digestion and overall well-being.

Case Study 2: Overcoming Candida Overgrowth with the Candida Diet:

- **Patient Background:** John, a 42-year-old man, faced recurrent yeast infections and digestive issues. He was diagnosed with Candida overgrowth.
- **Dietary Intervention:** John implemented the Candida diet, eliminating sugar and refined grains while incorporating anti-fungal foods.
- **Outcome:** John saw a marked improvement in his symptoms, including reduced yeast infections and improved digestive health. He also noted an increase in energy levels and overall vitality.

Conclusion:

Managing SIBO and Candida overgrowth requires a tailored dietary approach that addresses the specific needs of each condition. By adopting targeted diets such as the Low FODMAP or Specific Carbohydrate Diet for SIBO, and the Candida diet or anti-fungal diet for Candida overgrowth, individuals can achieve significant symptom relief and improve their digestive health. Real-life case studies highlight the effectiveness of these dietary strategies, demonstrating their potential to enhance well-being and quality of life. Implementing these protocols, with careful monitoring and adjustments, can lead to successful management of these challenging conditions.

Chapter 10
Gut-Brain Connection and Mental Health

I.   How Gut Health Affects Mental Health:

- ### The Gut-Brain Axis:

The gut-brain axis is a bidirectional communication network linking the central nervous system (brain) and the enteric nervous system (gut). This connection is facilitated through neural pathways (particularly the vagus nerve), hormonal signals, and immune system mediators. The health of the gut significantly impacts brain function and vice versa. For instance, stress and anxiety can affect gut motility and function, while gut health can influence mood and cognitive processes:

- ### Microbiome Influence on the Brain:

The gut microbiome consists of trillions of microorganisms that play a crucial role in maintaining overall health. These microorganisms produce neurotransmitters like serotonin (often called the "happy chemical"), dopamine, and GABA, which are essential for mood regulation and cognitive function. About 90% of the body's serotonin is produced in the gut, highlighting the significant impact of gut health on mental well-being. Dysbiosis, or an imbalance in the gut microbiome, can lead to altered neurotransmitter production, contributing to mental health issues such as anxiety and depression:

- ### Inflammation and Mental Health:

Chronic gut inflammation, caused by factors like poor diet, stress, and infections, can lead to increased intestinal permeability (commonly referred to as "leaky gut"). This condition allows toxins, undigested food particles, and pathogens to enter the bloodstream, potentially reaching the brain and triggering or exacerbating mental health disorders. Reducing gut inflammation through dietary and lifestyle changes can therefore have a positive impact on mental health:

II. Dietary Strategies to Support the Gut-Brain Axis:

• Probiotics and Mental Health:

Probiotics are live bacteria and yeasts that are beneficial for gut health. They can be found in fermented foods like yogurt, kefir, sauerkraut, and kimchi, or taken as supplements. Specific strains of probiotics, such as Lactobacillus and Bifidobacterium, have been shown to alleviate symptoms of anxiety and depression by enhancing gut health, reducing inflammation, and improving the production of beneficial neurotransmitters. Studies suggest that these probiotics can help restore balance in the gut microbiome, which is crucial for mental health:

• Prebiotics for a Healthy Microbiome:

Prebiotics are types of fiber that feed the beneficial bacteria in the gut. Foods rich in prebiotics include garlic, onions, leeks, asparagus, bananas, and whole grains. Consuming prebiotics promotes the growth of healthy gut bacteria, which can enhance the production of neurotransmitters and reduce inflammation. By supporting a balanced gut microbiome, prebiotics indirectly contribute to improved mood and cognitive function:

• Anti-Inflammatory Diet:

An anti-inflammatory diet can help reduce chronic inflammation in the gut, thereby supporting mental health. This diet includes a variety of fruits, vegetables, whole grains, lean proteins, and healthy fats. Omega-3 fatty acids, found in fatty fish (like salmon and mackerel), flaxseeds, chia seeds, and walnuts, are particularly beneficial due to their strong anti-inflammatory properties. Additionally, foods rich in antioxidants, such as berries, green tea, and dark chocolate, can help combat oxidative stress and inflammation, promoting both gut and brain health:

• **Avoiding Gut Irritants:**

Certain foods and substances can irritate the gut lining and contribute to inflammation and dysbiosis. These include highly processed foods, refined sugars, artificial sweeteners, and excessive alcohol. Gluten and dairy can also be problematic for some individuals, particularly those with sensitivities or intolerances. Minimizing or eliminating these irritants from the diet can help improve gut health, which in turn supports mental health:

III. **Mindfulness and Stress Reduction Techniques:**

• **Mindfulness Practices:**

Mindfulness involves focusing on the present moment and being aware of your thoughts, feelings, and bodily sensations without judgment. Regular mindfulness practices, such as meditation, deep breathing exercises, and yoga, can reduce stress and anxiety, which are known to negatively impact gut health. Mindfulness can help lower levels of the stress hormone cortisol, reduce gut inflammation, and improve symptoms of irritable bowel syndrome (IBS). Practicing mindfulness for even a few minutes each day can lead to significant improvements in both gut and mental health:

• **Stress Management:**

Chronic stress can alter gut motility, increase gut permeability, and disrupt the balance of the gut microbiome. Implementing effective stress management techniques is crucial for maintaining a healthy gut-brain axis. Regular physical activity, such as walking, swimming, or cycling, can help reduce stress and improve gut health. Additionally, ensuring adequate sleep, engaging in hobbies, and spending time with loved ones can help manage stress levels. Techniques such as progressive muscle relaxation, guided imagery, and biofeedback can also be effective in reducing stress and its impact on gut health:

- ## Cognitive Behavioral Therapy (CBT):

    CBT is a type of psychotherapy that helps individuals identify and change negative thought patterns and behaviors. It has been shown to be effective in treating both mental health disorders and gut-related issues like IBS. By addressing the psychological aspect of gut health, CBT can enhance overall well-being. For example, CBT can help individuals manage stress, anxiety, and depression, which in turn can improve gut symptoms. Working with a trained therapist can provide personalized strategies to manage both mental and digestive health:

- ## Practical Tips for Integrating Gut-Brain Health Strategies:

    ### Balanced Diet:

    Ensure your diet includes a variety of nutrient-dense foods that support both gut and brain health. Focus on incorporating plenty of fiber, probiotics, and prebiotics, and avoid processed and inflammatory foods. Aim to eat a rainbow of colorful fruits and vegetables, lean proteins, and healthy fats. Pay attention to portion sizes and try to eat meals at regular intervals to support digestive health:

    ### Regular Exercise:

    Physical activity is not only beneficial for overall health but also supports a healthy gut microbiome and reduces stress levels. Exercise promotes the growth of beneficial gut bacteria and can help regulate gut motility. Aim for at least 30 minutes of moderate exercise most days of the week, such as walking, jogging, swimming, or cycling. Incorporate strength training exercises to build muscle and improve overall fitness:

Adequate Sleep:

Prioritize good sleep hygiene by maintaining a regular sleep schedule, creating a restful sleep environment, and avoiding stimulants like caffeine before bedtime. Quality sleep is crucial for both gut and mental health. Aim for 7-9 hours of sleep per night, and establish a calming bedtime routine, such as reading, taking a warm bath, or practicing relaxation techniques:

Mindfulness and Relaxation:

Incorporate mindfulness practices into your daily routine. Even a few minutes of meditation or deep breathing exercises can significantly reduce stress and support the gut-brain connection. Consider setting aside time each day for mindfulness activities, such as mindful walking, yoga, or journaling. These practices can help you stay grounded and improve your overall well-being:

Hydration:

Stay well-hydrated by drinking plenty of water throughout the day. Proper hydration supports digestive health and helps maintain the integrity of the gut lining. Aim to drink at least 8 glasses of water per day, and consider increasing your intake if you are physically active or live in a hot climate. Herbal teas, such as chamomile or peppermint, can also support digestion and provide additional hydration:

Conclusion:

The gut-brain connection is a powerful link that plays a crucial role in overall health and well-being. By understanding the impact of gut health on mental health and implementing dietary strategies, mindfulness practices, and lifestyle changes, individuals can support both their gut and brain, leading to improved mood, reduced anxiety, and enhanced cognitive function. Fostering a healthy gut-brain axis is an essential component of holistic health care and can significantly enhance quality of life. Through conscious efforts to maintain gut health, one can experience profound benefits in mental and emotional well-being.

Chapter 11
Special Considerations: Children and Elderly

I. <u>Nutritional Needs for Different Age Groups:</u>

• <u>Children:</u>

Children's nutritional needs are crucial for their growth, development, and overall health. They require a balanced intake of macronutrients (carbohydrates, proteins, and fats) and micronutrients (vitamins and minerals) to support their rapidly developing bodies. Here are some key nutritional components and their sources:

- **Protein:** Essential for growth, repair, and immune function. Good sources include lean meats, poultry, fish, eggs, dairy products, beans, lentils, and tofu. Children typically need about 1 gram of protein per kilogram of body weight.
- **Calcium:** Vital for bone and teeth development. Sources include milk, cheese, yogurt, fortified plant-based milks, leafy green vegetables, and fortified cereals. The recommended daily intake varies with age but ranges from 700 mg to 1,300 mg.
- **Iron:** Necessary for cognitive development and oxygen transport in the blood. Sources include red meat, poultry, fish, beans, lentils, spinach, and iron-fortified cereals. Children aged 1-3 need about 7 mg per day, while those aged 4-8 need 10 mg.
- **Fiber:** Supports digestive health and regular bowel movements. Sources include fruits, vegetables, whole grains, and legumes. Children should consume about 19-25 grams of fiber per day.
- **Vitamins and Minerals:** A diverse diet ensures adequate intake of essential vitamins (A, C, D, E, and B-complex) and minerals (zinc, magnesium, potassium). Encourage a variety of colorful fruits and vegetables to meet these needs.

- **<u>Elderly</u>:**

As people age, their digestive systems and nutritional needs change. Elderly individuals may experience reduced digestive enzyme production, decreased nutrient absorption, and altered metabolism. Key dietary considerations include:

- **Protein:** To prevent muscle loss and support immune function. Good sources include lean meats, fish, eggs, dairy products, and plant-based proteins like beans and lentils. Older adults should aim for 1-1.2 grams of protein per kilogram of body weight.
- **Fiber:** To combat constipation and support overall digestive health. Sources include whole grains, fruits, vegetables, nuts, and seeds. The recommended daily intake is about 21 grams for women and 30 grams for men.
- **Calcium and Vitamin D:** To maintain bone health and reduce the risk of osteoporosis. Sources include dairy products, fortified plant-based milks, leafy greens, and supplements if necessary. The recommended daily intake for calcium is 1,200 mg, and for vitamin D, it's 800-1,000 IU.
- **Hydration:** Older adults are at higher risk of dehydration due to reduced thirst sensation and potential medication side effects. Encourage regular fluid intake through water, herbal teas, and hydrating foods like soups and fruits.
- **Small, Frequent Meals:** Eating smaller, more frequent meals can aid digestion and prevent discomfort, especially for those with diminished appetite or digestive issues.

II.   <u>Addressing Pediatric and Geriatric Digestive Issues:</u>

- **<u>Pediatric Digestive Issues:</u>**

Children can experience various digestive issues, including constipation, diarrhea, and food intolerances. Effective management involves specific dietary strategies and practical tips:

Constipation:

- **Dietary Fiber:** Increase fiber intake through fruits (apples, pears, berries), vegetables (carrots, broccoli, peas), and whole grains (oatmeal, whole-wheat bread, brown rice).
- **Hydration:** Ensure children drink plenty of water throughout the day.
- **Physical Activity:** Encourage regular physical activity to stimulate bowel movements.

Diarrhea:

- **Hydration:** Maintain hydration with oral rehydration solutions, water, and clear broths.
- **BRAT Diet:** Use the BRAT diet (bananas, rice, applesauce, toast) temporarily to ease digestion.
- **Probiotics:** Introduce probiotics through yogurt or supplements to restore healthy gut bacteria.

Food Intolerances:

- **Identification:** Work with a healthcare provider to identify trigger foods through elimination diets.
- **Management:** Eliminate identified trigger foods (such as lactose or gluten) and find suitable alternatives.
- **Education:** Educate the child and family about reading food labels and avoiding cross-contamination.

- ## Geriatric Digestive Issues:

Common digestive issues in the elderly include constipation, acid reflux, and reduced digestive enzyme production. Addressing these requires specific dietary and lifestyle adjustments:

Constipation:

- **Fiber Intake:** Increase fiber intake with high-fiber foods like prunes, bran, oatmeal, and fiber supplements if necessary.
- **Hydration:** Encourage regular fluid intake to soften stools.
- **Physical Activity:** Promote regular exercise such as walking, which can help stimulate bowel movements.

Acid Reflux:

- **Dietary Adjustments:** Avoid trigger foods such as spicy, fatty, and acidic foods. Eat smaller, more frequent meals.
- **Lifestyle Changes:** Avoid lying down immediately after eating, elevate the head of the bed, and maintain a healthy weight.
- **Medications:** Use antacids or other medications as prescribed by a healthcare provider.

Digestive Enzyme Insufficiency:

- **Enzyme Supplements:** Consider enzyme supplements (such as lactase or pancreatin) if recommended by a healthcare provider.
- **Easily Digestible Foods:** Focus on foods that are easier to digest, like steamed vegetables, lean proteins, and cooked fruits.

III.   <u>Practical Advice for Caregivers:</u>

- <u>**For Children:**</u>

    Caregivers play a crucial role in maintaining children's digestive health. Practical tips include:

    - **Balanced Meals:** Provide balanced meals that include a variety of food groups. Encourage children to eat a colorful array of fruits and vegetables, whole grains, and lean proteins.

- **Routine:** Establish regular meal and snack times to promote consistent digestion and prevent overeating.
- **Hydration:** Encourage water intake throughout the day and limit sugary drinks to prevent digestive issues and support overall health.
- **Positive Environment:** Create a positive eating environment free from distractions like TV or electronic devices. Encourage family meals to promote healthy eating habits.
- **Education and Involvement:** Involve children in meal planning and preparation to teach them about healthy eating and make them more likely to try new foods.

- **For Elderly:**

Caring for elderly individuals requires attention to their unique nutritional needs and digestive challenges. Tips for caregivers include:

- **Meal Planning:** Plan meals that are nutrient-dense and easy to digest. Include a variety of colorful fruits and vegetables, lean proteins, and whole grains.
- **Hydration:** Ensure regular fluid intake by offering water, herbal teas, and hydrating foods like soups and fruits with high water content.
- **Monitor Health:** Keep track of any digestive issues or changes in bowel habits and consult with healthcare providers as needed.
- **Adapt Meals:** Adjust the texture and consistency of foods if the elderly individual has difficulty chewing or swallowing. Soft, cooked foods, purees, and smoothies can be good options.
- **Encourage Activity:** Promote regular physical activity to aid digestion and overall health. Simple activities like walking or stretching can be beneficial.
- **Nutritional Supplements:** If necessary, incorporate nutritional supplements to ensure adequate intake of vitamins and minerals,

particularly if the elderly individual has a poor appetite or specific deficiencies.

Conclusion:

Maintaining digestive health is essential for both children and the elderly, as their nutritional needs and digestive challenges differ significantly from those of adults. By understanding these unique requirements and implementing tailored dietary and lifestyle strategies, caregivers can support the digestive health and overall well-being of these vulnerable age groups. Ensuring a balanced diet, proper hydration, and addressing specific digestive issues can lead to improved health outcomes and a better quality of life for both children and elderly individuals. Through attentive care and appropriate nutritional support, it is possible to foster optimal digestive health across all stages of life.

Chapter 12
Functional Foods and Supplements for Digestive Health

I. <u>Overview of Beneficial Supplements:</u>

• <u>Probiotics:</u>

Probiotics are live microorganisms that provide health benefits when consumed in adequate amounts. They help maintain a healthy balance of gut bacteria, which is crucial for digestive health. Common probiotic strains include Lactobacillus, Bifidobacterium, and Saccharomyces boulardii. These strains can be found in various supplements and fermented foods. Benefits of probiotics include:

- **Restoring Gut Flora:** Probiotics can replenish beneficial bacteria in the gut, especially after antibiotic use or gastrointestinal infections.
- **Reducing Symptoms of IBS:** Specific probiotic strains can help alleviate symptoms of irritable bowel syndrome (IBS), such as bloating, gas, and diarrhea.
- **Enhancing Immune Function:** Probiotics support the immune system by maintaining a balanced gut microbiome.

• <u>Prebiotics:</u>

Prebiotics are non-digestible fibers that act as food for beneficial gut bacteria. They help promote the growth and activity of these bacteria, contributing to a healthy gut environment. Common prebiotics include inulin, fructo-oligosaccharides (FOS), and galacto-oligosaccharides (GOS). Benefits of prebiotics include:

- **Improving Digestion:** Prebiotics enhance the growth of beneficial bacteria, which aid in the digestion and absorption of nutrients.

- **Supporting Gut Health:** By promoting a healthy balance of gut bacteria, prebiotics can help prevent digestive disorders and improve overall gut health.
- **Boosting Immune Function:** Prebiotics contribute to a strong immune system by supporting the growth of beneficial gut bacteria.

• Digestive Enzymes:

Digestive enzymes are proteins that help break down food into smaller, absorbable components. They are naturally produced by the body but can also be taken as supplements to aid digestion, especially in individuals with enzyme deficiencies. Common digestive enzymes include amylase (breaks down carbohydrates), protease (breaks down proteins), and lipase (breaks down fats). Benefits of digestive enzymes include:

- **Enhancing Nutrient Absorption:** By improving the breakdown of food, digestive enzymes help the body absorb nutrients more efficiently.
- **Reducing Digestive Discomfort:** Enzyme supplements can alleviate symptoms such as bloating, gas, and indigestion, especially after consuming difficult-to-digest foods.
- **Supporting Individuals with Enzyme Deficiencies:** People with conditions like lactose intolerance or pancreatic insufficiency can benefit from enzyme supplements to aid digestion.

• Fiber Supplements:

Fiber is essential for maintaining healthy digestion and regular bowel movements. While dietary fiber should primarily come from food sources, supplements can help individuals who have difficulty meeting their fiber needs through diet alone. Common fiber supplements include psyllium husk, methylcellulose, and wheat dextrin. Benefits of fiber supplements include:

- **Promoting Regular Bowel Movements:** Fiber adds bulk to stools and helps prevent constipation.
- **Supporting Gut Health:** Fiber feeds beneficial gut bacteria, promoting a healthy microbiome.
- **Managing Blood Sugar Levels:** Fiber can slow the absorption of sugar, helping to stabilize blood sugar levels.

II.   Functional Foods and Their Benefits:

• Fermented Foods:

Fermented foods are rich in probiotics, which support a healthy gut microbiome. Common fermented foods include yogurt, kefir, sauerkraut, kimchi, miso, and kombucha. Benefits of fermented foods include:

- **Improving Digestion:** Fermented foods enhance digestion by introducing beneficial bacteria that aid in the breakdown of food.
- **Boosting Immunity:** The probiotics in fermented foods support the immune system by maintaining a balanced gut microbiome.
- **Reducing Inflammation:** Fermented foods can help reduce gut inflammation and improve symptoms of digestive disorders like IBS.

• High-Fiber Foods:

Fiber is crucial for digestive health, and high-fiber foods help maintain regular bowel movements and prevent constipation. Common high-fiber foods include fruits (berries, apples, pears), vegetables (broccoli, carrots, leafy greens), legumes (beans, lentils), and whole grains (oats, quinoa, brown rice). Benefits of high-fiber foods include:

- **Promoting Regularity:** Fiber adds bulk to stools, making them easier to pass and preventing constipation.
- **Supporting Gut Health:** Fiber feeds beneficial gut bacteria, promoting a healthy balance of gut microbiota.

- **Lowering Cholesterol:** Soluble fiber can help reduce cholesterol levels by binding to cholesterol in the digestive system and preventing its absorption.

- **Omega-3 Fatty Acids:**

Omega-3 fatty acids are essential fats that have anti-inflammatory properties and support overall health. They can be found in fatty fish (salmon, mackerel, sardines), flaxseeds, chia seeds, and walnuts. Benefits of omega-3 fatty acids include:

- **Reducing Inflammation:** Omega-3s help reduce inflammation in the gut and other parts of the body, which can improve symptoms of inflammatory bowel disease (IBD) and other inflammatory conditions.
- **Supporting Heart Health:** Omega-3s can lower the risk of heart disease by reducing blood pressure, triglycerides, and cholesterol levels.
- **Improving Mental Health:** Omega-3s are beneficial for brain health and can help reduce symptoms of depression and anxiety.

- **Herbal Teas:**

Herbal teas can soothe the digestive system and support overall digestive health. Common herbal teas for digestion include peppermint, ginger, chamomile, and fennel. Benefits of herbal teas include:

- **Relieving Indigestion:** Peppermint and ginger teas can help relieve symptoms of indigestion, such as bloating and gas.
- **Calming the Stomach:** Chamomile tea has anti-inflammatory and calming properties that can soothe the digestive tract and reduce stomach cramps.
- **Supporting Regularity:** Fennel tea can help promote regular bowel movements and reduce bloating.

III. <u>Integrating Supplements into Daily Routines:</u>

- ### <u>Consulting Healthcare Providers:</u>

Before starting any new supplement regimen, it is important to consult with a healthcare provider. They can help determine the appropriate supplements based on individual health needs and conditions. This is particularly important for individuals with pre-existing health conditions or those taking medications, as some supplements can interact with medications or exacerbate certain conditions.

- ### <u>Consistency:</u>

To experience the benefits of supplements, consistency is key. Incorporate supplements into your daily routine by taking them at the same time each day. Setting reminders or using a pill organizer can help ensure regular intake.

- ### <u>Balanced Diet:</u>

Supplements should complement, not replace, a balanced diet. Aim to get the majority of nutrients from whole foods, using supplements to fill any gaps. A diet rich in fruits, vegetables, whole grains, lean proteins, and healthy fats provides a wide range of nutrients essential for digestive health.

- ### <u>Hydration:</u>

Adequate hydration is crucial for the effectiveness of fiber supplements and overall digestive health. Drink plenty of water throughout the day to support digestion and help fiber work effectively.

- ## <u>Monitoring and Adjusting:</u>

Regularly monitor your digestive health and overall well-being to assess the effectiveness of the supplements. Adjust dosages or switch to different products, if necessary, based on how your body responds. Working with a healthcare provider can help make informed decisions about any adjustments needed.

Conclusion:

Functional foods and supplements play a significant role in supporting and maintaining digestive health. By incorporating probiotics, prebiotics, digestive enzymes, and fiber supplements into your daily routine, you can enhance nutrient absorption, improve gut health, and reduce digestive discomfort. Additionally, functional foods such as fermented foods, high-fiber foods, omega-3 fatty acids, and herbal teas offer natural and effective ways to promote a healthy digestive system. Always consult with healthcare providers before starting any new supplements and focus on maintaining a balanced diet for optimal digestive health. Through mindful integration of these nutritional strategies, you can achieve and sustain a healthy and well-functioning digestive system.

Chapter 13
The Role of Lifestyle in Digestive Health

Digestive health is profoundly influenced by various lifestyle factors that extend beyond diet alone. This chapter delves into the multifaceted relationship between lifestyle choices and digestive health, exploring the impact of exercise, sleep, and stress management on the gastrointestinal system. By understanding and optimizing these factors, individuals can significantly improve their digestive health and overall well-being.

I.   <u>Impact of Exercise on Digestion:</u>

Regular physical activity plays a critical role in maintaining a healthy digestive system. Exercise stimulates intestinal contractions, which can help prevent constipation and promote regular bowel movements. Additionally, physical activity enhances blood flow to the digestive organs, supporting optimal function:

- **<u>Types of Exercise Beneficial for Digestion:</u>**
  - **Aerobic Exercise:** Activities like walking, jogging, swimming, and cycling increase heart rate and stimulate intestinal activity, aiding in digestion and reducing symptoms of bloating and constipation. Aerobic exercises improve cardiovascular health, which is closely linked to digestive efficiency. The increased oxygen flow helps in the optimal functioning of digestive organs:
  - **Strength Training:** Building muscle mass through resistance exercises can improve metabolism and support digestive health. Strength training exercises like weight lifting can enhance the body's overall metabolic rate, helping in more efficient digestion and nutrient absorption:
  - **Yoga and Stretching:** Specific yoga poses and stretching exercises can help relieve gas, reduce bloating, and promote a

healthy digestive tract. Poses such as twists, forward bends, and poses that involve core engagement can directly stimulate digestive organs and encourage the flow of digestive juices:

- **Exercise Recommendations:**
  - **Aerobic Activity:** Aim for at least 150 minutes of moderate aerobic activity or 75 minutes of vigorous activity per week, combined with muscle-strengthening activities on two or more days per week. Activities like brisk walking, running, swimming, or cycling are excellent choices:
  - **Strength Training:** Incorporate strength training exercises at least twice a week. Focus on major muscle groups and consider incorporating exercises like squats, lunges, push-ups, and weight lifting:
  - **Yoga and Stretching:** Integrate yoga or stretching sessions into your weekly routine. Even short, daily sessions can be beneficial. Poses like the seated twist, child's pose, and cat-cow stretch are particularly good for digestion:

II. Importance of Sleep and Stress Management:

Quality sleep and effective stress management are crucial for maintaining digestive health. Poor sleep and chronic stress can disrupt the digestive process, leading to various gastrointestinal issues such as irritable bowel syndrome (IBS), acid reflux, and indigestion:

- **The Sleep-Digestive Health Connection:**
  - **Sleep Patterns:** Consistent sleep patterns help regulate the body's circadian rhythms, which influence digestive function. Disruptions in sleep can lead to gastrointestinal discomfort and impaired digestion. The body performs many restorative functions during sleep, including those that affect digestion:

- **Sleep Position:** Sleeping on the left side can aid digestion and reduce acid reflux symptoms, as it allows gravity to assist in the natural downward movement of food and digestive juices. This position can prevent stomach acid from flowing back into the esophagus, reducing the likelihood of heartburn:

- **Stress and Its Impact on Digestion:**
  - **Stress Response:** The body's stress response, including the release of cortisol and adrenaline, can affect gut motility and increase the risk of digestive disorders. Chronic stress can alter the balance of gut bacteria, leading to conditions like IBS:
  - **Mind-Gut Connection:** The gut-brain axis highlights the bidirectional communication between the gut and the brain, where stress and anxiety can exacerbate digestive symptoms. Stress can lead to changes in gut motility, increased gut sensitivity, and alterations in gut microbiota:

- **Techniques for Improving Sleep and Reducing Stress:**
  - **Sleep Hygiene:** Maintain a regular sleep schedule, create a relaxing bedtime routine, and ensure a comfortable sleep environment. Practices such as avoiding screens before bedtime, keeping the bedroom dark and cool, and establishing a regular bedtime can improve sleep quality:
  - **Relaxation Practices:** Incorporate relaxation techniques such as deep breathing exercises, meditation, and progressive muscle relaxation to reduce stress levels. Practices like mindfulness meditation can lower cortisol levels and improve gut health:
  - **Mindfulness:** Practicing mindfulness and staying present in the moment can help alleviate stress and improve overall mental well-being. Mindfulness techniques can include mindful eating, where individuals focus on the sensory experience of eating, promoting better digestion:

III. <u>Creating a Holistic Lifestyle Plan:</u>

Integrating the principles of exercise, sleep, and stress management into a holistic lifestyle plan can significantly enhance digestive health. This comprehensive approach ensures that all aspects of an individual's life are aligned to support optimal gastrointestinal function:

- **<u>Steps to Develop a Holistic Lifestyle Plan:</u>**
  - **Assessment:** Begin by assessing current lifestyle habits, identifying areas for improvement in physical activity, sleep patterns, and stress management. Use tools like food diaries, sleep journals, and stress assessments to gather baseline data:
  - **Goal Setting:** Set realistic and achievable goals for incorporating regular exercise, improving sleep hygiene, and practicing stress-reduction techniques. Goals should be specific, measurable, achievable, relevant, and time-bound (SMART):
  - **Routine Establishment:** Create a daily and weekly routine that includes scheduled times for exercise, relaxation practices, and consistent sleep patterns. Consistency is key to forming lasting habits. Plan activities like morning walks, evening yoga sessions, and regular bedtime routines:
  - **Monitoring and Adjustment:** Regularly monitor progress and make necessary adjustments to the plan to ensure continued improvement in digestive health and overall well-being. Keep track of symptoms, progress towards goals, and adjust strategies as needed to stay on track:

Conclusion:

A holistic approach to lifestyle can have a profound impact on digestive health. By integrating regular exercise, quality sleep, and effective stress management into daily life, individuals can significantly improve their digestive function and overall health. This chapter underscores the importance of a comprehensive, multifaceted approach to achieving and maintaining optimal digestive wellness:

Chapter 14
Personalizing Dietary Therapies

Personalizing dietary therapies is crucial for effectively managing digestive health issues. Each individual has unique dietary needs based on their specific health conditions, genetic makeup, lifestyle, and personal preferences. This chapter explores how clinicians can assess individual needs, customize diet plans for different conditions, and monitor and adjust dietary interventions to achieve optimal digestive health.

I. <u>Assessing Individual Needs:</u>

Understanding the specific needs of each patient is the first step in personalizing dietary therapies. This involves a thorough assessment of the patient's health history, current symptoms, lifestyle, and dietary habits:

- **Health History:**

A detailed health history should include information about the patient's past and present digestive issues, family history of digestive disorders, and any other relevant medical conditions. This helps in identifying potential genetic predispositions and underlying causes of digestive problems.

  - **Medical Conditions:** Assess for comorbid conditions like diabetes, cardiovascular diseases, or autoimmune disorders that might influence digestive health.
  - **Medications:** Consider the impact of any medications the patient is taking, as some drugs can affect digestion and nutrient absorption:
  - **Surgical History:** Evaluate any previous gastrointestinal surgeries that might affect digestive function.

- **Symptom Diary:**

Encourage patients to keep a diary of their symptoms, noting the time, frequency, and severity of each episode. This can help in identifying patterns and potential triggers, providing valuable insights for developing a personalized diet plan:

- **Frequency of Symptoms:** Track how often symptoms occur to determine if they are related to specific foods, activities, or times of day.
- **Severity and Duration:** Assess the severity and duration of symptoms to understand the impact on the patient's quality of life.
- **Context:** Note any contextual factors, such as stress levels or recent dietary changes, that might influence symptoms.

- **Lifestyle Assessment:**

Evaluate the patient's lifestyle, including physical activity levels, stress factors, sleep patterns, and daily routines. Understanding these aspects is essential for creating a comprehensive and practical dietary plan:

- **Physical Activity:** Determine the type, frequency, and intensity of physical activity, as exercise can significantly influence digestion.
- **Stress Levels:** Assess the patient's stress levels and coping mechanisms, as chronic stress can exacerbate digestive issues.
- **Sleep Patterns:** Evaluate sleep quality and patterns, as poor sleep can negatively affect digestive health.

- **Dietary Habits:**

Assess the patient's current diet, including food preferences, eating habits, and any known food intolerances or allergies. A detailed food diary can be particularly helpful in this process, highlighting areas that need adjustment:

- **Macronutrient Balance:** Evaluate the balance of carbohydrates, proteins, and fats in the patient's diet.
- **Meal Timing and Frequency:** Assess the timing and frequency of meals and snacks, as irregular eating patterns can affect digestion.
- **Hydration Status:** Consider the patient's fluid intake, as proper hydration is essential for digestive health.

II. <u>Customizing Diet Plans for Different Conditions:</u>

Different digestive health conditions require tailored dietary approaches. Here, we discuss specific dietary strategies for managing some common digestive disorders.

- **<u>Irritable Bowel Syndrome (IBS):</u>**
  - **Low FODMAP Diet:** A low FODMAP (Fermentable Oligosaccharides, Disaccharides, Monosaccharides, and Polyols) diet can be highly effective for managing IBS symptoms. This diet involves avoiding high-FODMAP foods that are poorly absorbed in the small intestine and can cause gas, bloating, and diarrhea.
  - **High-FODMAP Foods:** Include foods like certain fruits (apples, pears), vegetables (onions, garlic), dairy products, and legumes:
  - **Phased Approach:** Implement the diet in phases – elimination, reintroduction, and maintenance – to identify specific triggers.

  - **Fiber Management:** Balancing fiber intake is crucial. Soluble fiber, found in foods like oats, apples, and carrots, can help regulate bowel movements, while insoluble fiber may need to be limited if it exacerbates symptoms.
  - **Soluble Fiber:** Helps in forming a gel-like substance in the intestines, slowing digestion and promoting stool formation:
  - **Insoluble Fiber:** Adds bulk to the stool but can cause irritation in sensitive individuals.

- **Hydration:** Adequate hydration is important, as it helps maintain normal bowel function and can alleviate constipation, a common issue in IBS.
- **Fluid Types:** Include water, herbal teas, and clear broths while avoiding caffeine and alcohol, which can irritate the gut.

- **Inflammatory Bowel Disease (IBD):**
  - **Anti-Inflammatory Diet:** Focus on foods that reduce inflammation, such as fatty fish (rich in omega-3 fatty acids), fruits, vegetables, whole grains, and nuts. Avoid foods that may trigger inflammation, such as processed foods, refined sugars, and saturated fats.
  - **Omega-3 Fatty Acids:** Found in salmon, mackerel, flaxseeds, and walnuts, these can help reduce inflammation.
  - **Antioxidant-Rich Foods:** Include berries, leafy greens, and nuts to combat oxidative stress and inflammation.
  - **Specific Carbohydrate Diet (SCD):** The SCD eliminates complex carbohydrates that are difficult to digest and can contribute to gut dysbiosis. This diet emphasizes simple, natural foods that are easier on the digestive system.
  - **Allowed Foods:** Include meat, fish, eggs, vegetables, and certain fruits:
  - **Avoided Foods:** Exclude grains, dairy, processed foods, and certain legumes.
  - **Nutritional Supplements:** Patients with IBD often have nutrient deficiencies due to malabsorption. Supplements like vitamin D, calcium, iron, and B vitamins may be necessary to address these deficiencies.
  - **Iron:** Essential for preventing anemia, common in IBD patients:
  - **Vitamin D and Calcium:** Important for bone health, particularly if corticosteroids are used in treatment.

- **Gastroesophageal Reflux Disease (GERD):**
  - **Trigger Foods:** Identify and avoid foods that trigger acid reflux, such as spicy foods, fatty foods, chocolate, caffeine, alcohol, and acidic foods like tomatoes and citrus fruits.
  - **Fatty Foods:** Slow down stomach emptying and relax the lower esophageal sphincter.
  - **Spicy Foods:** Can irritate the esophagus and increase acid production.
  - **Meal Timing:** Encourage patients to eat smaller, more frequent meals instead of large meals, and to avoid eating at least three hours before bedtime to reduce the risk of nighttime reflux.
  - **Portion Control:** Smaller meals reduce the pressure on the stomach and esophageal sphincter:
  - **Timing:** Avoid lying down immediately after meals to prevent reflux.
  - **Weight Management:** Maintaining a healthy weight can significantly reduce GERD symptoms. Excess weight puts pressure on the abdomen, pushing stomach contents up into the esophagus.
  - **Weight Loss Strategies:** Incorporate gradual and sustainable weight loss methods, focusing on a balanced diet and regular physical activity.

III. Monitoring and Adjusting Dietary Interventions:

Continuous monitoring and regular adjustments are vital to the success of personalized dietary therapies. Here's how to effectively manage and adjust dietary plans:

- **Regular Follow-Ups:** Schedule regular follow-up appointments to monitor the patient's progress, discuss any new symptoms or challenges, and make necessary adjustments to the diet plan.
- **Frequency:** Depending on the severity of the condition, follow-ups can range from weekly to monthly.
- **Evaluation:** Use follow-ups to assess adherence to the diet, symptom improvement, and overall well-being.

- **Patient Feedback:** Encourage patients to provide feedback about how they feel on their new diet. This can include any improvements in symptoms, energy levels, and overall well-being.
- **Open Communication:** Create a supportive environment where patients feel comfortable discussing their experiences and challenges.
- **Feedback Tools:** Utilize surveys, symptom trackers, and digital apps to gather detailed feedback.
- **Dietary Adjustments:** Based on the patient's feedback and progress, make incremental adjustments to the diet. This could involve reintroducing certain foods, increasing or decreasing specific nutrients, or trying new dietary strategies.
- **Reintroduction Phase:** Gradually reintroduce eliminated foods to identify specific triggers.
- **Nutrient Optimization:** Adjust macronutrient and micronutrient intake to meet the patient's changing needs.
- **Education and Support:** Educate patients about the importance of adherence to their personalized diet and provide support through educational materials, cooking tips, and access to nutrition counseling.
- **Resources:** Provide handouts, recipes, and online resources tailored to the patient's dietary plan.
- **Support Groups:** Encourage participation in support groups for shared experiences and encouragement.

Conclusion:

Personalizing dietary therapies is a dynamic and ongoing process that requires a thorough understanding of the patient's unique needs, careful planning, and continuous monitoring. By tailoring diet plans to address specific digestive health conditions and individual preferences, clinicians can help patients achieve better digestive health and overall wellness. This chapter highlights the importance of a personalized approach to dietary therapies, ensuring that each patient receives the most effective and appropriate care for their digestive health needs.

Chapter 15
Recipes and Meal Plans for Digestive Health

Introduction:

In this chapter, we delve into the practical application of the nutritional strategies discussed throughout the book. We provide a comprehensive collection of recipes and meal plans designed to support digestive health. Whether you are managing conditions like IBS, GERD, or IBD, or simply aiming for optimal gut health, these recipes are tailored to meet various dietary needs while promoting a balanced and enjoyable eating experience. By incorporating these recipes into your daily routine, you can effectively support your digestive system and overall well-being.

I.   Easy-to-Follow Recipes:

• Breakfast Recipes:

1. Gut-Soothing Smoothie:

▪ Ingredients:

1 cup unsweetened almond milk.

1 ripe banana.

1/2 cup blueberries.

1 tablespoon chia seeds.

1/2 teaspoon ground ginger.

▪ Instructions:

Combine all ingredients in a blender.

Blend until smooth.

Serve immediately.

- **Benefits:** This smoothie is rich in fiber, antioxidants, and anti-inflammatory compounds, making it gentle on the gut and supportive of digestive health.

2. Oatmeal with Flaxseeds and Berries:

- **Ingredients:**

  1/2 cup rolled oats.

  1 cup water or milk of choice.

  1 tablespoon ground flaxseeds.

  1/2 cup mixed berries.

  1 tablespoon honey (optional).

- **Instructions:**

  Cook the oats in water or milk according to package instructions.

  Stir in ground flaxseeds.

  Top with mixed berries and honey if desired.

  Serve warm.

- **Benefits:** Oats and flaxseeds provide soluble fiber, which aids in digestion and helps maintain bowel regularity.

- **Lunch Recipes:**

1. Quinoa and Vegetable Salad:

- **Ingredients:**

  1 cup cooked quinoa.

  1/2 cup diced cucumber.

  1/2 cup cherry tomatoes, halved.

1/4 cup red bell pepper, diced.

2 tablespoons chopped fresh parsley.

2 tablespoons olive oil.

Juice of 1 lemon.

Salt and pepper to taste.

- **Instructions:**

In a large bowl, combine cooked quinoa, cucumber, tomatoes, bell pepper, and parsley.

Drizzle with olive oil and lemon juice.

Season with salt and pepper.

Toss to combine.

Serve chilled.

- **Benefits:** This salad is high in fiber and antioxidants, promoting a healthy gut environment and reducing inflammation.

2. Chicken and Avocado Wrap:

- **Ingredients:**

1 whole-grain tortilla.

1/2 cup cooked, shredded chicken breast.

1/4 avocado, sliced.

1/4 cup shredded lettuce.

1/4 cup grated carrots.

2 tablespoons hummus.

- **Instructions:**

Spread hummus on the tortilla.

Layer with chicken, avocado, lettuce, and carrots.

Roll up the tortilla tightly.

Slice in half and serve.

- **Benefits:** This wrap provides lean protein, healthy fats, and fiber, supporting a balanced and gut-friendly meal.

- **Dinner Recipes:**

1. Baked Salmon with Asparagus:

- **Ingredients:**

2 salmon fillets.

1 bunch asparagus, trimmed.

2 tablespoons olive oil.

1 lemon, sliced.

Salt and pepper to taste.

- **Instructions:**

Preheat oven to 400°F (200°C).

Place salmon fillets and asparagus on a baking sheet.

Drizzle with olive oil and season with salt and pepper.

Top with lemon slices.

Bake for 15-20 minutes, until salmon is cooked through and asparagus is tender.

- **Benefits:** Salmon is rich in omega-3 fatty acids, which reduce inflammation, while asparagus provides prebiotics to nourish beneficial gut bacteria.

2. Vegetable Stir-Fry with Tofu:

- ### Ingredients:

  1 block firm tofu, cubed.

  1 tablespoon sesame oil.

  1 cup broccoli florets.

  1 red bell pepper, sliced.

  1 carrot, julienned.

  2 tablespoons soy sauce or tamari.

  1 tablespoon grated ginger.

  2 cloves garlic, minced.

- ### Instructions:

  Heat sesame oil in a large pan over medium heat.

  Add tofu cubes and cook until golden brown on all sides.

  Add broccoli, bell pepper, and carrot, and stir-fry for 5-7 minutes.

  Stir in soy sauce, ginger, and garlic.

  Cook for an additional 2-3 minutes.

  Serve over brown rice or quinoa.

- **Benefits:** This stir-fry is packed with fiber, vitamins, and minerals, and tofu provides a plant-based protein source that is easy on the digestive system.

- ### Snack Recipes:

1. Yogurt with Honey and Walnuts:

- ### Ingredients:

  1 cup plain Greek yogurt.

1 tablespoon honey.

1/4 cup chopped walnuts.

- ■ **Instructions:**

Spoon yogurt into a bowl.

Drizzle with honey and top with walnuts.

Serve immediately.

- **Benefits:** Greek yogurt contains probiotics that support gut health, while honey and walnuts add prebiotics and healthy fats.

2. Carrot and Cucumber Sticks with Hummus:

- ■ **Ingredients:**

1 large carrot, cut into sticks.

1 cucumber, cut into sticks.

1/2 cup hummus.

- ■ **Instructions:**

Arrange carrot and cucumber sticks on a plate.

Serve with a side of hummus for dipping.

- **Benefits:** This snack is rich in fiber and healthy fats, supporting digestion and providing a satisfying and nutritious option.

II.   **Weekly Meal Plans:**

- **Meal Plan for IBS:**

Monday:

Breakfast: Gut-Soothing Smoothie

Lunch: Quinoa and Vegetable Salad

Snack: Yogurt with Honey and Walnuts

Dinner: Baked Salmon with Asparagus

Tuesday:

Breakfast: Oatmeal with Flaxseeds and Berries

Lunch: Chicken and Avocado Wrap

Snack: Carrot and Cucumber Sticks with Hummus

Dinner: Vegetable Stir-Fry with Tofu

Wednesday:

Breakfast: Gut-Soothing Smoothie

Lunch: Quinoa and Vegetable Salad

Snack: Yogurt with Honey and Walnuts

Dinner: Baked Salmon with Asparagus

Thursday:

Breakfast: Oatmeal with Flaxseeds and Berries

Lunch: Chicken and Avocado Wrap

Snack: Carrot and Cucumber Sticks with Hummus

Dinner: Vegetable Stir-Fry with Tofu

Friday:

Breakfast: Gut-Soothing Smoothie

Lunch: Quinoa and Vegetable Salad

Snack: Yogurt with Honey and Walnuts

Dinner: Baked Salmon with Asparagus

Saturday:

Breakfast: Oatmeal with Flaxseeds and Berries

Lunch: Chicken and Avocado Wrap

Snack: Carrot and Cucumber Sticks with Hummus

Dinner: Vegetable Stir-Fry with Tofu

Sunday:

Breakfast: Gut-Soothing Smoothie

Lunch: Quinoa and Vegetable Salad

Snack: Yogurt with Honey and Walnuts

Dinner: Baked Salmon with Asparagus

- **<u>Meal Plan for GERD:</u>**
  Monday:

  Breakfast: Gut-Soothing Smoothie

  Lunch: Chicken and Avocado Wrap

  Snack: Carrot and Cucumber Sticks with Hummus

  Dinner: Baked Salmon with Asparagus

Tuesday:

Breakfast: Oatmeal with Flaxseeds and Berries

Lunch: Quinoa and Vegetable Salad

Snack: Yogurt with Honey and Walnuts

Dinner: Vegetable Stir-Fry with Tofu

Wednesday:

Breakfast: Gut-Soothing Smoothie

Lunch: Chicken and Avocado Wrap

Snack: Carrot and Cucumber Sticks with Hummus

Dinner: Baked Salmon with Asparagus

Thursday:

Breakfast: Oatmeal with Flaxseeds and Berries

Lunch: Quinoa and Vegetable Salad

Snack: Yogurt with Honey and Walnuts

Dinner: Vegetable Stir-Fry with Tofu

Friday:

Breakfast: Gut-Soothing Smoothie

Lunch: Chicken and Avocado Wrap

Snack: Carrot and Cucumber Sticks with Hummus

Dinner: Baked Salmon with Asparagus

Saturday:

Breakfast: Oatmeal with Flaxseeds and Berries

Lunch: Quinoa and Vegetable Salad

Snack: Yogurt with Honey and Walnuts

Dinner: Vegetable Stir-Fry with Tofu

Sunday:

Breakfast: Gut-Soothing Smoothie

Lunch: Chicken and Avocado Wrap

Snack: Carrot and Cucumber Sticks with Hummus

Dinner: Baked Salmon with Asparagus

III.   **Tips for Meal Preparation and Planning:**

- **Batch Cooking:**
  - Prepare large quantities of grains like quinoa, rice, and oats at the beginning of the week. Store them in airtight containers for quick access.
  - Cook proteins such as chicken, tofu, or fish in bulk and portion them out for different meals.

- **Pre-Cutting Vegetables:**
  - Wash, peel, and cut vegetables in advance. Store them in the refrigerator so they are ready to use for salads, stir-fries, and snacks.
  - Use resealable bags or containers to keep them fresh.

- **Utilize Leftovers:**
  - Repurpose leftovers from dinner for lunch the next day. For example, use leftover baked salmon in a salad or wrap.

- Combine different leftovers to create new meals and reduce food waste.

- **<u>Meal Planning:</u>**
  - Plan your meals for the week ahead. This helps ensure you have all necessary ingredients and reduces the likelihood of making unhealthy food choices.
  - Create a grocery list based on your meal plan to streamline your shopping and avoid impulse buys.

- Mindful Eating:
  - Eat slowly and chew your food thoroughly. This aids in digestion and allows you to savor your meals.
  - Avoid distractions like TV or smartphones during meals to focus on your food and recognize your body's hunger and fullness signals.

Conclusion:

Incorporating these recipes and meal plans into your daily routine can significantly enhance your digestive health. By focusing on nutrient-dense, gut-friendly foods, you can alleviate symptoms of common digestive disorders and support overall wellness. Remember, consistency is key. Regularly consuming these balanced meals will help maintain a healthy digestive system and promote long-term health benefits.

Conclusion

- ### <u>Conclusion of the Book:</u>

In conclusion, "Dietary Therapies for Digestive Health: A Clinician's Handbook" serves as a comprehensive guide to understanding and improving digestive health through proven nutritional strategies. Throughout this handbook, we have delved into various aspects of digestive health, ranging from the anatomy and functions of the digestive system to practical dietary interventions for managing common disorders such as IBS, GERD, and IBD.

- ### <u>Recap of Key Topics:</u>

1. Understanding Digestive Health:

- We began by exploring the anatomy and importance of the digestive system, emphasizing its role in nutrient absorption and overall well-being.

2. The Gut Microbiome:

- We discussed the critical role of the gut microbiome in digestion and its impact on immune function, mental health, and disease prevention.

3. Dietary Interventions:

- Detailed dietary approaches were provided for managing conditions like irritable bowel syndrome (IBS), Inflammatory Bowel Disease (IBD), and Gastroesophageal Reflux Disease (GERD), emphasizing the role of fiber, hydration, and specific dietary restrictions.

4. Elimination Diets and Food Sensitivities:

- We explored the importance of identifying food intolerances and implementing elimination diets to alleviate digestive symptoms.

5. Fiber and Hydration:

- The benefits of dietary fiber and adequate hydration were highlighted for maintaining digestive regularity and supporting gut health.

6. Nutritional Strategies:

- Strategies for managing constipation, diarrhea, and integrating fermented foods and beneficial supplements were discussed to optimize digestive function.

7. Lifestyle Factors:

- We emphasized the impact of exercise, sleep, stress management, and a holistic lifestyle plan on digestive health.

8. Personalized Dietary Approaches:

- The importance of assessing individual needs and customizing diet plans based on specific conditions or preferences was underscored.

9. Recipes and Meal Plans:

- Practical recipes and meal plans were provided to demonstrate how to incorporate gut-friendly foods into daily eating habits, promoting digestive wellness.

Detailed Results

Certainly! Here are detailed and expanded results derived from "Dietary Therapies for Digestive Health: A Clinician's Handbook:"

➤ **<u>Comprehensive Understanding of Digestive Health:</u>**
- Readers gain a thorough comprehension of the digestive system, encompassing its anatomical structure, physiological functions, and the crucial role it plays in overall health and disease prevention.
- Detailed insights into the digestive process, including nutrient absorption, enzymatic actions, and the interplay between different organs such as the stomach, small intestine, and colon.

➤ **<u>Effective Management of Digestive Disorders:</u>**
- The handbook provides evidence-based dietary interventions tailored for managing a spectrum of digestive disorders:
- Irritable Bowel Syndrome (IBS): Strategies include low-FODMAP diets, fiber supplementation, and identifying trigger foods.
- Inflammatory Bowel Disease (IBD): Focuses on anti-inflammatory diets, omega-3 fatty acids, and avoiding specific food groups that exacerbate symptoms.
- Gastroesophageal Reflux Disease (GERD): Emphasizes dietary modifications to reduce acid reflux, such as avoiding spicy foods, caffeine, and fatty meals.
- Case studies and success stories illustrate practical applications of these strategies, showcasing real-life improvements in symptom management and quality of life.

➤ **<u>Optimization of Gut Microbiome Health:</u>**
- Detailed exploration of the gut microbiome's significance in digestion, immune function, and overall health.

- Strategies for enhancing microbiome diversity through probiotics, prebiotics, and fermented foods, promoting a balanced gut environment crucial for digestive health.
- Practical guidance on incorporating probiotic-rich foods like yogurt, kefir, and fermented vegetables into daily diets to support beneficial gut bacteria.

➢ **<u>Practical Guidance on Elimination Diets and Food Sensitivities:</u>**
- Comprehensive methods for identifying food intolerances and implementing elimination diets to pinpoint trigger foods contributing to digestive discomfort.
- Step-by-step protocols for reintroducing eliminated foods to identify specific sensitivities, aiding in long-term management of conditions like lactose intolerance or gluten sensitivity.

➢ **<u>Promotion of Dietary Fiber and Hydration:</u>**
- In-depth exploration of dietary fiber types (soluble vs. insoluble) and their respective roles in digestive health, including promoting regular bowel movements and supporting gut microbiome health.
- High-fiber meal plans and recipes designed to increase fiber intake naturally through whole grains, fruits, vegetables, and legumes.
- Importance of adequate hydration in maintaining digestive regularity and facilitating optimal nutrient absorption, with practical hydration tips and herbal teas beneficial for digestive wellness.

➢ **<u>Integration of Lifestyle Factors:</u>**
- Holistic approach addressing the impact of lifestyle factors on digestive health, including:

- Exercise: Benefits of regular physical activity in promoting gastrointestinal motility and reducing symptoms of constipation.
- Sleep: Importance of adequate sleep for gut microbiome balance and overall digestive function.
- Stress Management: Techniques such as mindfulness, relaxation exercises, and stress reduction strategies to alleviate stress-related digestive symptoms.

> **<u>Personalized Approaches to Diet and Nutrition:</u>**
- Guidance on assessing individual dietary needs based on specific digestive conditions, genetic factors, and personal preferences.
- Customizable diet plans tailored to address varying severity levels and stages of digestive disorders, empowering individuals to optimize their nutrition for symptom management and long-term health.

> **<u>Empowerment Through Practical Tools:</u>**
- Practical tools including recipes, meal plans, and shopping lists that facilitate implementation of recommended dietary strategies.
- Case studies and success stories illustrating the efficacy of dietary therapies in real-life scenarios, empowering readers with actionable insights and motivation for adopting healthier eating habits.

> **<u>Holistic Approach to Wellness:</u>**
- Emphasis on the interconnectedness of diet, lifestyle, and mental health in achieving comprehensive digestive wellness.
- Encouragement of a holistic lifestyle approach that supports not only symptom management but also overall health optimization and disease prevention.

> ### **Long-Term Health Benefits:**
- By adopting the strategies outlined in the handbook, individuals can experience sustained improvements in digestive function, reduced reliance on medications, and enhanced quality of life.
- Potential long-term benefits include reduced risk of chronic digestive disorders, improved immune function, and overall well-being through proactive management of digestive health.

In conclusion, "Dietary Therapies for Digestive Health: A Clinician's Handbook" equips readers with in-depth knowledge, practical tools, and personalized strategies to achieve optimal digestive health. By integrating these insights into daily routines, individuals can proactively manage digestive disorders, promote gut microbiome health, and enhance overall well-being effectively.

www.ingramcontent.com/pod-product-compliance
Lightning Source LLC
Chambersburg PA
CBHW061059250726
48653CB00001B/465